fork it

Keys To Amazing Health

SUZANNE MILES

black card
B O O K S

Author: Suzanne Miles
Title: Fork It
ISBN: 978-1-77204-196-5
Category: HEALTH & FITNESS/Diet & Nutrition/General

Publisher:
Black Card Books
Division of Gerry Robert Enterprises Inc.
Suite 214, 5-18 Ringwood Drive
Stouffville, Ontario
Canada, L4A 0N2
International Calling: 1 647 361 8577
www.blackcardbooks.com

fork it
Keys To Amazing Health

SUZANNE MILES

black card
B O O K S

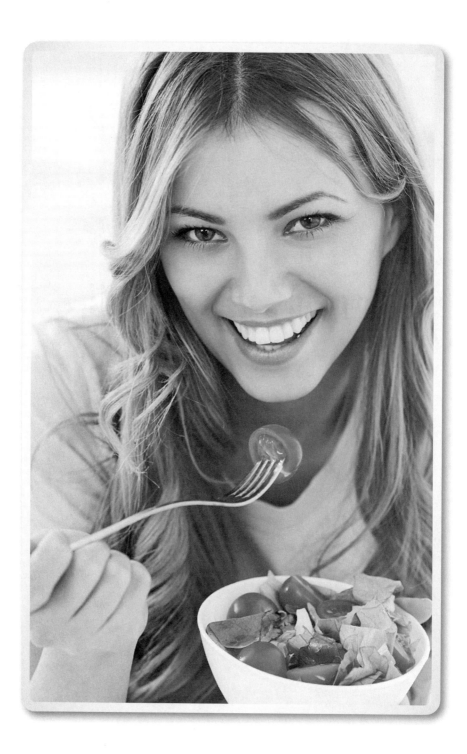

Table Of Contents

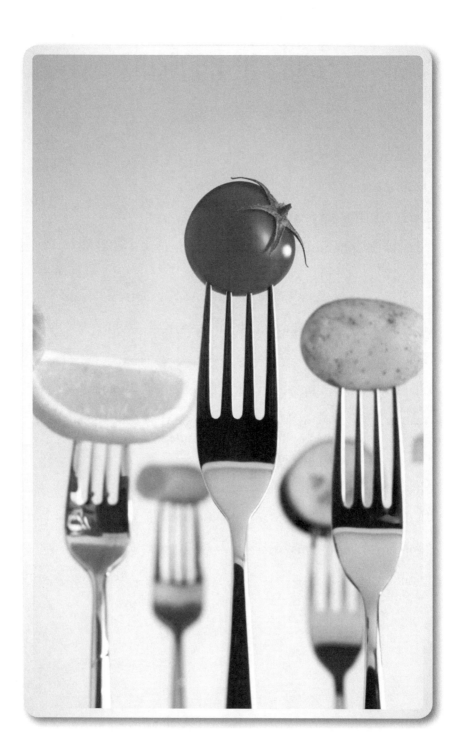

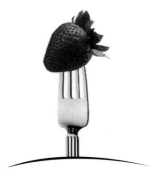

ABOUT THE AUTHOR

Suzanne Miles

*S*uzanne Miles lives with her husband and business partner, Tony Norrish, in the picturesque mountains of North Vancouver, British Columbia, Canada. She is a food researcher and author with a keen interest in motivating people to achieve amazing health. Suzanne is interested in inspiring people by raising awareness of how food choices directly impact your health. Suzanne is committed to making a positive difference in the health of people, the freedom of animals and the care of the environment everywhere.

Suzanne's research led her to become a practicing vegan in 2011 at the age of 54. Her continuing research and practical methods have garnered her worldwide recognition. Her personal achievements include weight loss, amazing health and increased vitality.

Suzanne enjoys an international lifestyle and has had a lifelong interest in natural health and healing remedies for physical, spiritual, and emotional well-being. Suzanne holds a Diploma of Health and Fitness from Shaw Academy in the UK, and have completed the Terry Willard course.

Fork It: Keys To Amazing Health, Suzanne's first book, is intended to inspire, motivate, and inform the reader about how the positive choices you make with food have a beneficial impact on your health and longevity.

Come along with Suzanne as she gives you inspiration and knowledge and shares practical, personal experiences that you can take with you to enjoy amazing health and reach your goals and dreams for a higher quality of life.

"Vegan, the gift that keeps on giving."

—SUZANNE MILES

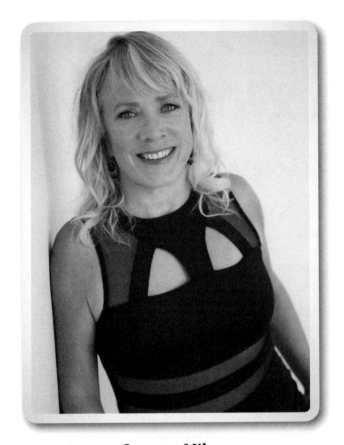

Suzanne Miles
Author
Fork It: Keys To Amazing Health

Website
www.forkitbook.com

Email
smiles00@live.com

Facebook
www.tinyurl.com/fork-it-Facebook
www.tinyurl.com/FB-SuzanneMiles

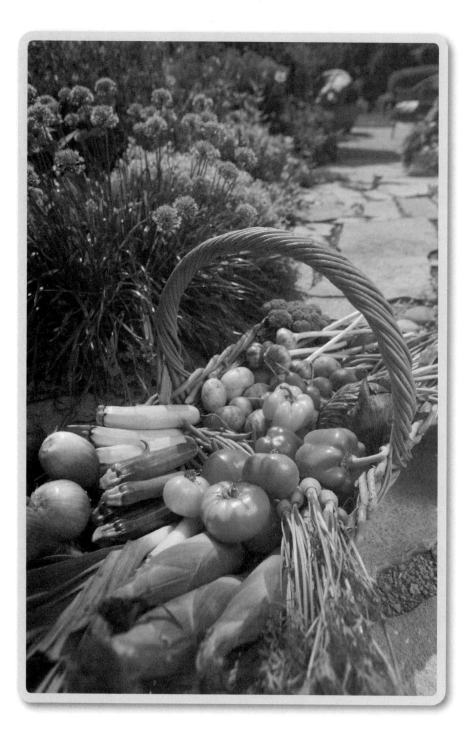

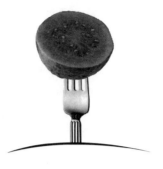

Dedication

I dedicate this book to my husband, Tony, for his instant willingness to switch to plant-based living together with me, hand in hand. Tony embraced the changes with all my meals and made many adjustments willingly and happily. Tony has given his own special touches to our plant-based lifestyle, embracing unique ways with food and food presentation.

Also to my amazing daughter, Leah, of whom I am very proud. She has an incredible inner strength and loving light that she brings to the world.

And to Tara, Tony's daughter, affectionately known as Baby Bear, who came to live with us at age fifteen. She embraced the vegan lifestyle with a discipline and dedication like one beyond her years.

To my cat, Sonya, whom I love very much. She thanks me every day with purrs and funny shows for being vegan and not eating any more of her friends.

My family, Tony, Leah, and Tara, have helped me to learn so much about myself and the benefits of plant-based living. They have been the ones tasting many new finds of foods, and the creations of the meals, juices, smoothies finding them all amazingly flavorful and delicious.

Vegan, plant-based living is the wave of the future, and I especially and always dedicate this book to people of all ages everywhere seeking keys to amazing health in harmony with our earth.

I especially dedicate this book to the children and animals of the future, who deserve excellent health and harmony on a home called earth.

Made with Love,

Suzanne Miles

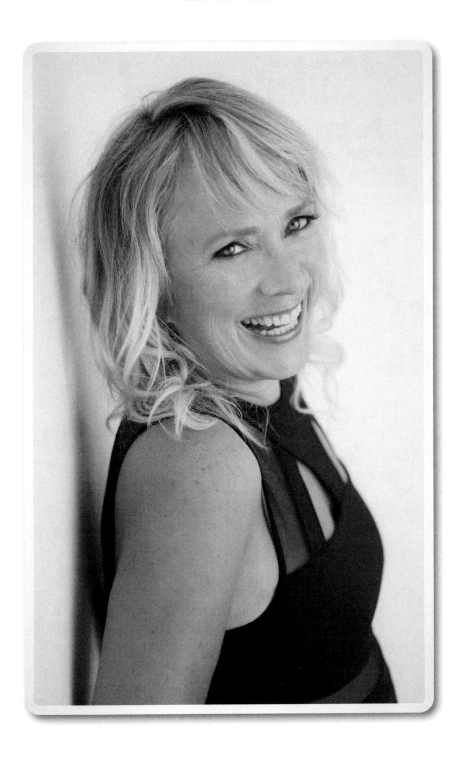

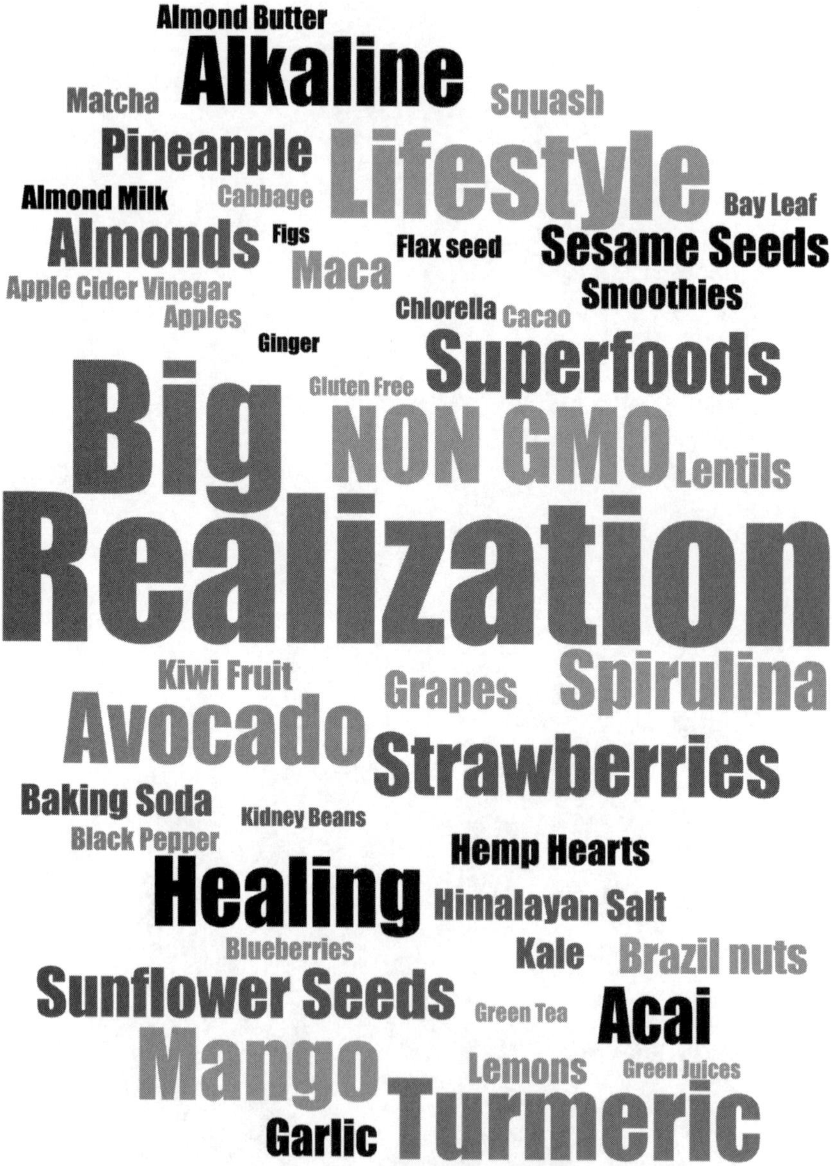

Almond Butter
Alkaline
Squash
Matcha
Pineapple
Lifestyle
Almond Milk Cabbage
Bay Leaf
Almonds Figs
Flax seed
Sesame Seeds
Apple Cider Vinegar
Maca
Smoothies
Apples
Chlorella Cacao
Ginger
Superfoods
Gluten Free
Big
NON GMO
Lentils
Realization
Kiwi Fruit
Grapes
Spirulina
Avocado
Strawberries
Baking Soda
Kidney Beans
Black Pepper
Hemp Hearts
Healing Himalayan Salt
Blueberries
Kale Brazil nuts
Sunflower Seeds Green Tea Acai
Mango Lemons Green Juices
Garlic Turmeric
Tomatoes Bok Choy
Arugula

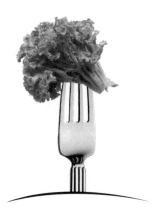

CHAPTER ONE

The Big Realization

*S*ummer of 2011. My doctor had sent me for the second time to consult with a surgeon about an internal issue regarding my health. I had been having this growth in me for about five years at that point. It was big, and I spent a lot of time dressing to hide it. I tried everything to reduce this beast in me, including exercise and vitamins, visits to the naturopath, acupuncture, sugar reduction, fast-food reduction; but still there it was—it wouldn't move. I don't even know where it came from, why it was there, or what it was. My question was, how can I defeat this growth and why is it that I have this internal issue anyway?

I was told surgical intervention was looking to be the only solution. The surgeon was just doing her job. So I asked her, "What's with this thing in me?"

She replied, "Well, it's neither gotten smaller nor has it grown; it's just kind of there."

I said, "So will YOU do the surgery?"

She said, "YES!" like this was a happy moment.

It was in the surgeon's office that I had an epiphany right in front of her. I said, "You know, with all due respect, I'm leaving now. This isn't my journey or my story—one of major surgery and a lifetime of pills with potential for emotional upheavals due to the hormone shake-up that may occur with this surgery," and I left.

I called my husband and I said to him, "We have to have everything organic, including meat, cheese, eggs, etc. All meats in particular have to be organic." The summer rolled on. Then in August 2011 I saw the advertisement for an upcoming documentary from Dr. Sanjay Gupta called *The Last Heart Attack*, and we set course to make sure we watched that show.

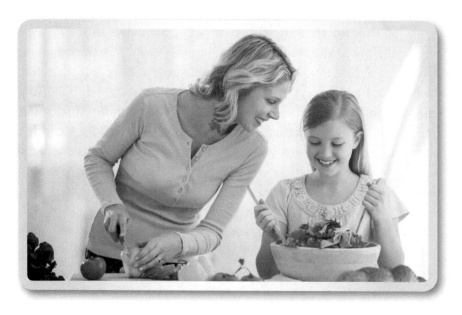

You see, prior to the summer of 2011, we thought we ate well. Although I was carrying weight heading towards 180+ pounds, my husband was heading towards 200 pounds. We had made many positive adjustments to our lifestyle and diet—or so we thought. I had been through ten years of learning that I had high cholesterol, that I was becoming an at-risk person for a heart attack, that my weight was increasing, that I should take the Healthy Heart Program at the local hospital, (which I did take); that I should take more fish oils, have tests for this and for that, and take statins, which thankfully I always refused and held that pressure at bay. It was all revolving around the doctor and tests, with talks about what the future might look like, and it wasn't a bright picture.

Finally, the documentary we had scheduled to watch arrived. It was a game changer. *The Last Heart Attack* by Dr. Sanjay Gupta featured Bill Clinton and Dr. Caldwell B. Esselstyn, an American surgeon, along with an incredible story of how Bill Clinton and many others interviewed took back their total health on a plant-based, vegan diet without any animal products, fat, or oils.

Immediately we decided to join the plant-based vegan revolution, at least to lose some weight. We cleared out our entire kitchen of everything. We looked with sharp eyes at every can of food, every box of everything, every cereal, every vitamin—everything got our total scrutiny, and 95 percent of what was in our kitchen went out the door.

I survived!!! I've survived since 2011 without eating any animal products. That means I've lived without cheese, yogurt, cottage cheese, pork, beef, chicken, lamb, eggs, fish, or any animals from the ocean, and that includes shrimp, oysters, crab and lobster. I also lived without sausages, roasts, ham, salami, and all those deli meats. I lived without meat pies and sausage rolls, pizza, bacon, milk, sour cream, cream, **I survived!!!** butter, or margarine. Oh yes, I almost forgot,

I also lived without wheat, gluten, GMO, alcohol, bread, pastries, cake, cookies, ice cream, chocolate bars and candy. Nothing deep-fried, and no trans-fat oils. Did I leave anything out? Oh yes, I lived without turkey for Thanksgiving and without turkey for Christmas. I lived without candy on Halloween and without chocolates on Valentine's Day. I lived without flowers (another heavily toxic item), chocolates, or expensive animal-based meals for my birthday. No more BBQs, no more fast-food on the run when we were out. I've lived without toxic detergents and body cleansers such as shampoo and conditioners, deodorant, and skin care products of all sorts. I also let go of the vitamin industry at this time because I couldn't feel any results. I was not alone on this path. I did this hand in hand with my husband and both our daughters, who at the time were fifteen and 25 years of age when we started.

We started our lives over on August 30, 2011. I was 54, and my husband was 57.

Right away we came across some challenges when we went to a social gathering and were offered a beautiful platter of cheeses and deli meats. We said no, and that was the beginning of our newfound discipline and life-changing empowerment, with one simple word with two letters, no, and of course, thank you!

Quickly we started to see more inspiring people who are living the plant-based, vegan way, including Ellen DeGeneres. She spoke in her interview with Katie Couric in March 2010 (see links in book), where she offered some great nuggets about why she doesn't eat animals, including the disconnect with food and the animals that share our planet. It was from Ellen that we first heard about the documentary *Earthlings*.

We were also fortunate early in our journey to come across Mimi Kirk who won, at age 71, The Sexiest Vegan of the Year Award from PETA, which launched her into the media and garnered much attention. Mimi Kirk is still vegan, traveling and speaking around the world looking even more youthful and amazing now, several years later. At the time of this writing she just turned 76 and is touring Europe with her plant-based, vegan message.

> **We never starved—we never went hungry.**

We started to shop for food differently, realizing that we couldn't go to the same stores we used to. We never starved—we never went hungry. We went through our fall and an entire winter in this transition. The gym became our friend. It was cold and raining, and we went every night for a speed walk or an elliptical run along with a sauna and a weigh-in at the scale on the way out. We took no classes, just that cardio, but each time we went, we gave it all we had.

After about three weeks, we noticed our weight beginning to show results in the way we wanted. This was very encouraging. Then around the fourth week it started; every time we stepped on the scale we were half a pound lighter, and this went on for another two weeks and then it stopped and stabilized for a period of 10–14 days. We just kept doing what we were doing, and after about two weeks, the weight loss started again at half a pound per day. We found these results to be extremely motivating to stay the course.

In between all this, we went through some peak periods of festive occasions in which traditional meals at gatherings were served. To our surprise, we were shocked that these meals were based around dead animals, and loaded with animal fat, butter, salt, sugar for desserts, and stuffing of organ meat; not to mention the alcohol libations that are customary as well, e.g., table wine, beer, and port after dinner.

Now we were delighted that our willpower and ever-strengthening discipline sustained us through challenging times. Still, we stayed the vegan and gym course. Why? Because we were getting results, and nothing was going to stop us now.

In the New Year, visits to the doctor showed levels starting to stabilize—a fantastic reward for our ability to stay with our newfound discipline. Eventually, my doctor said, "Whatever you're doing, keep doing it!" which was a miracle because also the fibroid was shrinking for the first time in ten years.

In the early days we noticed our energy level improve, weight drop, skin tone improve, and our discipline was further bolstered.

Eventually, we noted that our sweat didn't smell after the gym, nor in day to day activities (we had stopped using deodorant). And the topic most people don't talk about, but should, is our daily stool became soft and easy to release. This was a miracle! We did spend about four months at the beginning, much to our surprise, releasing incredible amounts of stored gas from the colon; but eventually that went away too. The stool became soft and easy as the body cleansed itself—as the miraculous machine that it is—of stored toxins and nasties from the old days of eating animal flesh and animal products.

In summary, after going through the first eight months of transition, we were inspired at how our bodies were cleaner and our weight was coming off. We were feeling highly energized, and the excitement of finding new foods and learning about new nutritional sources has been an awesome culinary adventure, full of options and information with exciting new flavours. We really enjoy shopping for our new food and coming home to make all kinds of new things. Our world of food expanded greatly at this time.

We thought we knew a lot, but this was exciting stuff!

A few keys we learned:

1. Stay with it, and don't buckle under pressure for any reason.

2. Shop in smaller stores where you can talk to the owners.

3. Find vegan restaurants that serve dishes you wouldn't otherwise think of making.

4. Always be changing up your food and improving on getting more raw foods in; eventually, you'll get there.

5. Remove toxins from your home, your body, and your life.

6. Understand that everyone won't be a fan of your journey, and they won't be coming with you. But new friends are waiting to meet you.

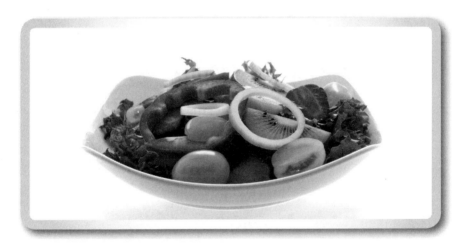

- Interview with Ellen DeGeneres on being vegan: www.tinyurl.com/Ellen-DeGeneres-on-being-vegan.

- Interview with Mimi Kirk on winning Sexiest Vegan of the Year, August 9, 2011: www.tinyurl.com/72-year-old-vegan-Mimi-Kirk.

- Dr. Sanjay Gupta's documentary, *The Last Heart Attack*: www.tinyurl.com/Dr-Sanjay-Gupta-documentary.

Bay Leaf

Almond Butter Flax seed Squash

Almond Milk

Almonds Pineapple Cacao Smoothies

Apple Cider Vinegar Matcha Sesame Seeds

Apples Cabbage Lentils Alkaline

Mango Maca Chlorella

Superfoods

Gluten Free Ginger

NON GMO Lifestyle

VEGAN

Figs

Kiwi Fruit Grapes Spirulina

Avocado Strawberries

Baking Soda Kidney Beans

Black Pepper Hemp Hearts

Acai Garlic Himalayan Salt

Blueberries Kale Brazil nuts

Sunflower Seeds Green Tea Healing

Arugula Lemons Green Juices

Tomatoes Turmeric

Bok Choy

8

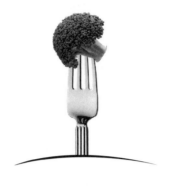

Congratulations - You're A Vegan

Throughout the first eight months, we went through quite a few phases as we kept adjusting to the many changes coming at us. Food was changing rapidly at this point as we started to let go of the "other way." Back then we ate tempeh and tofu, and grilled vegan cheese and soy sauce. We had tried alternative sausages and gluten-free bread. We were still frying in oil as much as we were practicing with juicing.

It was around this eight-month point that we realized just how far we'd come with our health. We all came out of winter with marked health improvements. This was an exciting time and my husband and I lost twenty pounds each. Bonus!!!

We were excited to start looking at new food ideas with the advent of spring and summer. We packed away most of the foods we'd been eating and working on through the winter, such as grilled cheese with gluten-free bread, vegan style; miso soups; we'd had some stir-fries and rice, and we'd had some juicing and some shakes, but mostly we'd tried to mimic the other way, the way we'd come from. It was time to let that go. Now we started to eat differently again, experimenting with more raw foods as the weather warmed up and our energy was much stronger.

By now our bodies had fallen into a nice biorhythm of improved cardio workouts and staying vegan. We'd seen some nice weight loss, and learned to bring in new foods. We felt stronger and faster because of less weight, less aches and pains, more health, more vibrancy, and continuing signs of improvement. Our confidence was building. We started to find new ways to reward ourselves for our discipline. We noticed that our cooking had changed quite a lot. It was always delicious, as we made everything from scratch. This was a big change

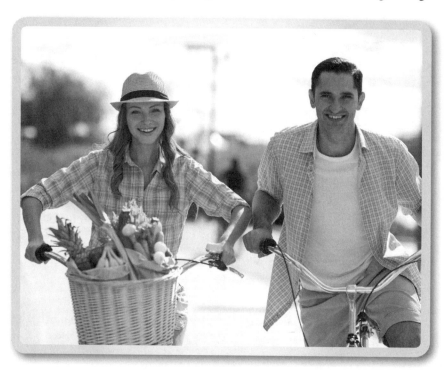

from the quicker-faster-sicker system we were once involved in. That summer, we took to more activities like trail running; hiking more; longer, quicker, faster walks; and much more cycling. We just started to spend a lot more time outdoors enjoying our newfound weight loss and fitness.

Still, the weight ebbed and flowed. Sometimes I'd put on five pounds, but by this point I would feel it, and I wasn't on the scale as frequently, so I knew my body better. I could feel my body more. I never worried about these things anymore. Instead, I just kept doing what I was doing. I stayed the course, and soon enough the five pounds melted away again.

You see, at the eight-month point, we had learned so much more that now we started counting chemicals, not calories. We started having more juices, more experiments with eating raw foods, while continuing to learn more about industrialized foods and their inherent dangers, while finding more organic foods and their inherent benefits.

People would say, "Wow, you look great! What are you doing?" or, "You've been vegan for how long?" or, "Gee, you've lost some weight, what are you doing?"

One of the key psychological elements that we learned throughout the process was not to allow ourselves to become hungry to the point that in the urgency to satisfy the hunger, we would make a poor food choice. One of our solutions to this situation was to carry a small container of dehydrated fruits, such as pineapple, figs, prunes, banana,

> . . . not to allow ourselves to become hungry to the point that in the urgency to satisfy the hunger, we would make a poor food choice.

and also a small assortment of nuts such as walnuts, almond, sunflower seeds, Brazil nut, goji berry, dates, and pumpkin seeds. I created a Grazing Drawer in the kitchen comprised of nine jars filled with a variety of healthy, organic, dehydrated fruits and assorted nuts and other goodies. This is still a popular drawer in our home today.

Right now I have dried prunes, pineapple, figs, sunflower and pumpkin seeds, mulberries, almonds, walnuts, watermelon seeds, and assorted nuts, including cashews, in the Grazing Drawer.

At this time we also discovered the wonders of dehydrated foods, including kale chips, crackers, bananas, dates, apricots, mulberries, kiwi, mango, and apple, to name a few. Then came in the nut butters such hemp butter, sesame butter, almond butter, and cashew butter. I also made my own nut milks. It was also at this time that the superfoods, herbs, and spices really came forward. Turmeric, cayenne, ginger, and cumin. We also learned much more about shopping for our food. Now we were buying in bulk at local farmers markets and small independent stores. It was in these places that items like dandelion leaves, burdock root, turmeric root, organic garlic, kukicha tea, spaghetti squash, spirulina, maca powder, chlorella, and wheat grass came into our lives big time.

In your first year of this transition, you start to have many epiphanies, or AH-HAs based on socially preconceived notions on many topics.

One of the enlightening concepts we stumbled upon during the first year was the mental paradigm shift that occurred. We spent our whole lives thinking that if the food is for sale in the stores, any food, it has to be safe to eat. But that's not true! We are eating chemicals!! Our society is currently seeing the greatest health risks ever, en masse, in our world. Chemicals and sugar are used for shelf life, binding agents, artificial flavourings and sweeteners. Clever words and heavy marketing disguise them. We have a global health epidemic of disease right now. Once you have built the foundation of plant-based living, and your house is solid, you really start questioning the entire system that you thought was safe. Your level of scrutiny rises such that you say no to eating anything that has a face or a mother, and even no to a birthday cake or a Mars bar or a Starbucks or a Baskin-Robbins ice cream. You won't do it anymore and congratulations, you're a vegan.

Being overweight is a direct result of your food choices and where you shop for your food. The foods of the system we once ate in are filled with chemicals that directly impact your body negatively at an alarming and cellular level. Most of this food is of

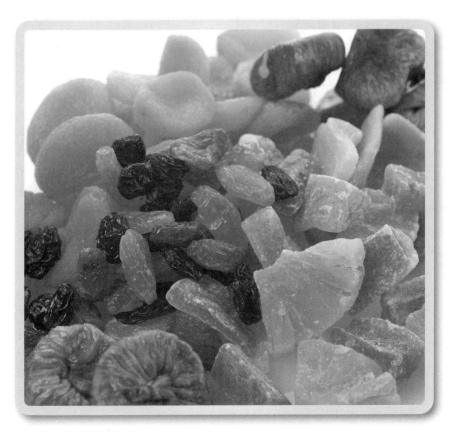

little to no nutrition value. In many circumstances, food developers have replaced farmers. Food developers are chemists!! Farmers and chemists are two different things!

The epiphany was that all this "dis-ease" we see everywhere in our society—and we were part of it—is a direct result of the food system. That means all the anti-aging pills, lotions, potions, all the vitamins, the skin care, the balding, the dry skin, the acne, the wheat belly, the many diseases of our modern society, are directly a result of food. Much of our food is genetically modified, especially in the United States where this is a serious, ongoing problem. We have been told a story about eating animals and the benefits of eating them that's not true—it's a story.

> The epiphany was that all this "dis-ease" we see everywhere in our society—and we were part of it—is a direct result of the food system.

The combination of the socially accepted way of thinking, combined with the fatty, high-salt, high-sugar, high-chemical, commercially mass-produced food products, along with diseased animals used as food, results in weight gain and a system of ill health in your body at a cellular level. This is the rise of dis-ease. It's moved us from plants for health to a sick system of disease and profit.

Once you close in on the one-year anniversary of being vegan, this is a time for a celebration. You have achieved and learned so much. It's a very gratifying journey as you enjoy your morning warm lemon drink and daily dose of apple cider vinegar or your green drink, knowing you are now in a position of empowerment for your life. The old, industrialized system seems so broken now as you view it from a distance.

Clearly, when you give your body a chance to cleanse, cleanse it does. Your body is an amazing machine. Give it a chance to clean up from the inside and it will respond quickly and noticeably, if you stay with the discipline. The key is to cleanse your organs. It's all about the inside. What you eat must feed your organs, not your stomach.

> *"Ask yourself what you can do for your body, and give your body a chance to show what it can do. It will respond either way. The human body is an amazing machine of balance."*
>
> —TONY NORRISH

When I was growing up, I had never heard of high blood pressure, cancer of every part of the body, multiple sclerosis, ADHD, and diabetes. All the kids of my generation—we were lean! If you were fat, you were one of a kind, not the norm. For example, in 1969, before fast-foods and McDonald's, the most famous music event was held—Woodstock. I highly recommend you watch the film, because there you will notice in over half a million people gathered in one place, very few, if any, are overweight.We never heard about these modern diseases. They have grown out of the industrial food system.

So, back to plants. You have to check out Mimi Kirk. She's a blonde beauty from San Diego who won at age 71 the Sexiest Vegan of the Year Award. She won it in the age group over 50, but she was 71. She is now 76 and on her European tour at the time of writing.

Your body is an amazing machine.

15

Here is a link to one of the interviews with Mimi Kirk upon winning this award: www.tinyurl.com/Mimi-Kirk-Sexy-Vegan.

Being vegan isn't just about eating salads and lettuce and carrots specifically. People may say you eat like a bird, or you eat like a rabbit, but that gets boring pretty quickly, and it's far from true.

At this one-year point you have embraced the vegan lifestyle, and you've probably bought a lot of new products, especially plant produce, and are trying new things. You may or may not have already discovered the other food groups that go hand in hand with the vegan lifestyle, and indeed, now is an opportunity to start letting go of some of the old products you were using and embrace cleaner, leaner ones.

These can include:

- Rice tortilla for making wraps
- Gluten-free foods
- Chickpea miso instead of soy for excellent soups and soup stocks
- Beans and legumes—kidney beans, chickpeas, lima beans, mung beans, red lentils, brown lentils, dried yellow and green peas
- Dandelion leaves, burdock root, romaine lettuce, yams, sweet potatoes
- Spices—turmeric, cumin, black pepper, Himalayan salt, saffron, cayenne, cardamon, ginger, saffron
- Goji berries, dried mission figs, medjool dates, hemp hearts
- Garlic and lemons
- Organic coconut oil
- Nut butters—hemp, cashew, sesame, almond, pumpkin butters

At this point you start to notice the difference in how you feel after you finish a meal. You remember how a year ago your meal was primarily comprised of meats, starch, chicken, fish, wine, beer, deli meats, bread, ice cream, and only a few vegetables. You had a sensation then of heaviness and immobility, such that you felt you needed a pick-me-up like a cup of coffee to re-start your energy after a meal.

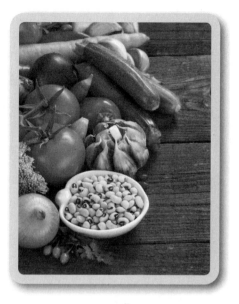

Now you notice after eating a meal of fresh vegetables and some legumes, beans, and spices that you feel energized after the meal, such that there is no need for a stimulus like coffee to kick-start your energy levels again. Instead, you may enjoy a nice cup of tea, perhaps green, chamomile, mint, and a brisk walk. You are no longer a couch potato—those days are gone. The TV is off.

This is a quantum shift and a feel-good difference. It's noticeable, and you start to strut. You're not going back to the old ways. You've just got started. New stores, new food ideas, cleaner food, more raw, more close to the source of the plant. You ask more questions now. You also start to remove toxins in your home at this point, but that's for another chapter.

With reduced weight and an energized feeling your activity levels increase, giving you the rewards of your newfound lifestyle.

Almond Butter Squash
Pineapple Lifestyle
Almond Milk Cabbage Bay Leaf
Almonds Figs Flax seed Sesame Seeds
Apple Cider Vinegar Maca Smoothies
Apples Chlorella Cacao
Ginger Superfoods
Gluten Free
Alkaline NON GMO Lentils

DEFENSE

Kiwi Fruit Grapes Spirulina
Avocado Strawberries
Baking Soda Kidney Beans
Black Pepper Hemp Hearts
Healing Himalayan Salt
Blueberries Kale Brazil nuts
Sunflower Seeds Green Tea Acai
Mango Lemons Green Juices
Garlic Turmeric
Tomatoes Bok Choy
Arugula

18

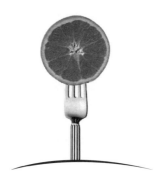

A Hidden Secret Exposed (Or A Secret Line Of Defense For Optimal Health)

*I*n my social encounters since becoming a vegan, I come across people who are curious and unsure about the word vegan. It confuses many. Not everybody knows really what this word means and it challenges them accordingly, because it's new information they don't understand.

As is true with most people when they are confronted with something new, they immediately refer to their ways of indoctrinated belief. It's very difficult to challenge the system you've been taught. People who are unwell look to the doctors and medications for cures instead of looking at their whole lifestyle for answers.

"Hidden from public information since the research first came out in 1931 is the case for the Alkaline Body, as the body that carries no disease, whereas the Acidic Body is the root cause of the all the cancers and disease. This acidic body is the true state of the word dis-ease."

—The Alkaline Body

As such, I came across the same questions many times from many people. "Oh, you're a vegan and your food is entirely plant-based? Really?" The most popular question following this comment is: "Where do you get your protein?" Another common question is: "How do you know you're getting enough amino acids?" Others say: "You can't rely on carbohydrates." Still others are very curious and ask, "How do you live on just plants?" A common misconception is that a plant-based diet is having a salad for breakfast, a salad for lunch, and another salad for dinner, and they assume all salads are the same. However, as many vegans will tell you, not all salads are the same.

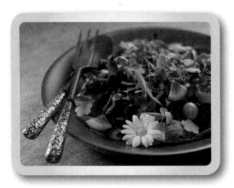

These questions led me to research for myself so that I could give answers to all these people who seemed to have these questions, including my immediate family, friends, and others I ran into as I went about my day.

I found this acidic body type topic to be curious because the research was leading to the fact that an acidic body is one that causes the state of disease, whereas an alkaline body is one of health. An acidic body is the cause of cancer, while an alkaline body state is one of health.

> **An acidic body is one that causes the state of disease, whereas an alkaline body is one of health.**

As I was researching the answers to these questions, it became apparent that 90% of Westernized people on our "industrialized food system" have acidic bodies. In the film *The Last Heart Attack* by Sanjay Gupta, featuring Bill Clinton, there was an interview with Dr. Caldwell B. Esselstyn, who discusses the plant-based vegan diet as the key to transitioning your body to a healthy pH balanced state, therefore avoiding not only heart disease but a plethora of other health problems.

This led me to a huge discovery about the work of Dr. Otto Heinrich Warburg:

"With a doctorate of chemistry, and a second doctorate in medicine, he was a physiologist and noted biochemist born in 1883 in Freiburg, Baden, Germany. Dr. Warburg won the Nobel Prize in Physiology or Medicine in 1931, and died in Berlin in 1970. He believed in eating organic."

"Dr. Warburg was awarded the Nobel Prize for his discovery that cancer is caused by weakened cell respiration due to lack of oxygen at the cellular level, and proving cancer thrives in anaerobic (without oxygen), or acidic, conditions. In other words, the main cause for cancer is acidity of the human body. In his Nobel Prize-winning study, Dr. Warburg illustrated the environment of the cancer cell. According to Warburg, damaged cell respiration causes fermentation, resulting in low pH (acidity) at the cellular level. Warburg also wrote about oxygen's relationship to the ph of cancer cells' internal environment. Since fermentation was a major metabolic pathway of cancer cells, warburg reported that cancer cells maintain a lower pH, as low as 6.0, Due to lactic acid production and elevated CO_2 He proved cancer cannot grow nor develop in body alkalinity of 7.36. He firmly believed that there was a direct relationship between ph and oxygen. Higher pH means higher concentration of oxygen molecules while lower pH means lower concentrations of oxygen. A normal healthy cell undergoes an adverse change when it can no longer take in oxygen to convert glucose into energy. In the absence of oxygen, the cell reverts to a primal nutritional program to nourish itself by converting glucose through the process of fermentation. The lactic acid produced by fermentation lowers the cell pH (acid/alkaline balance)

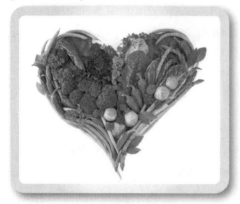 and destroys the ability of DNA and RNA to control cell division. The cancer cells then begin to multiply. The lactic acid simultaneously causes severe local pain as it destroys cell enzymes. Cancer appears as a rapidly growing external cell covering, with a core of dead cells."

So we have known the proven cause, prevention, and cure of cancer since 1931.

Dr. Otto Warburg finished one of his most famous speeches, "The Prime Cause and Prevention of Cancer", with the following statement: "…nobody today can say that one does not know what cancer and its prime cause is. On the contrary, there is no disease whose prime cause is better known, so that today ignorance is no longer an excuse that one cannot do more about prevention."

Considering fats to be the main contributor to weight gain is a popular misconception that leads to massive confusion, and explains why so many overweight people are not succeeding in losing weight. Many people would be shocked to find out that we may gain weight from eating cheese not only because it is rich in fat, but mostly due to its high acidic level. In response to high pH acid, the body creates fat cells to store the acid. Almonds have 70% fat, and pork has only 58%. However, pork has one of the highest acid values, -38, while almonds are alkaline forming, +3. Cucumbers and watermelons are so alkalizing that they can neutralize the acidifying effect of eating beef. This is why it is very important to know the pH index of all foods, showing the food's ability to alkalize the body. Please see the reference links to pH Food Indexes.

> ... it is very important to know the pH index of all foods, showing the food's ability to alkalize the body.

The so-called "bad" cholesterol, lipoprotein (LDL), is made by our own liver in order to bind the toxins and deactivate the acidic waste that came from certain food, not to cause arteriosclerosis (3).

Food, stress, mood, and music all alter our pH balance. Anything that is stimulating could leave an acidic residue in our body; any activities that are calming and relaxing could make us more alkaline. Dr. Caldwell believes 80% or more of cancers are initiated by or caused by STRESS, which alters our pH balance, which makes us acidic.

A lack of education about dietary pH balance results in confusion among people who are trying to eat healthy and stay alkaline to lose weight and to avoid cancer. Test your pH with litmus paper, and you will discover on days you eat leafy greens (kale, collards, Swiss chard, etc.) you will be healthily alkaline; on the days you don't, you won't be alkaline, even if you're eating raw. Here is the pH test strip paper[1] I use:

Once cancer has gained a foothold, it does not survive well in the presence of an alkaline cellular pH level, nor in the presence of highly oxygenated cells. As Nobel Laureate Otto Warburg discovered, low cellular oxygen is a primary causal factor for cancer. Perhaps you have heard the name Dr. Joanna Budwig, or *The Budwig Protocol.* Dr. Johanna Budwig of Germany, who passed away in 2003, was Dr. Warburg's protégé in 1951. She continued Dr. Warburg's work and

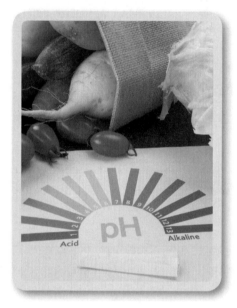

found that in order for proper cellular utilization of oxygen to take place, our diets must contain adequate amounts of unsaturated fatty acids. Over a fifty-year period, Johanna Budwig had a medically documented 90%-plus cancer cure rate in Germany with 4,500 patients. Some cancer victims that she cured with her protocol were considered terminal. See reference link #5 below if interested in more information on *The Budwig Protocol.*

Source 1: "The Prime Cause and Prevention of Cancer." Dr. Otto Warburg lecture delivered to Nobel Laureates on June 30, 1966 at Lindau, Lake Constance, Germany. www.stopcancer.com/ottolecture3.htm

---

1   www.tinyurl.com/sparkpeoplepublicjournal

Right now you are asking yourself, "Do I have an alkaline or an acidic body, and how do I find this out?"

How To Test Your pH

Your pH can be measured using a simple at-home test that measures the acidity of your urine (first of the day is best) or saliva. Instructions on how to use them come with the test; they are simple and easy to understand, so we recommend them as you begin the process of switching to an alkaline diet. The first step in establishing an alkaline diet is to assess your current pH. A good approximation of tissue pH is easily obtained by testing the pH of your saliva or first-morning urine. Follow these simple steps to test your pH at home;

1. Obtain and become familiar with the pH test paper included in your kit. This paper measures the acid-alkaline state of any liquid. Readings at the low end of the scale indicate an acidic state, and those on the higher end a more alkaline state.

2. First thing in the morning, preferably after six hours of sleep, get a test strip or tear off a three-inch piece of paper from the roll.

    a. Testing with urine: Either urinate directly on the paper, or collect urine in a cup and dip the paper into the urine in the cup. Please note that first-morning urine (after six hours of sleep without urinating) is the most valuable pH reading according to our research.

    b. Testing with saliva (if you can't go six hours without urinating): Rinse your mouth with water, spit it out into the sink, and spit again. Now, collect some saliva in a spoon and moisten the paper in the saliva. Do not eat, drink, or brush your teeth before the test.

3. As the test paper is moistened, it will take on a color. The color relates to the acid or alkaline state of your urine or saliva, and ranges from yellow to dark blue. Match the color of your test strip with the chart provided on the back of your test kit. A number below seven means that your urine is on the acid side. The lower the number, the more acidic the condition. Seven indicates a neutral state, neither acid nor alkaline.

4. The ideal urine reading should be between 6.5 to 7.5, and saliva readings should be between 7.0 to 7.5, with an occasional lower (more acidic) reading. Below, we give you tips on what to do if your reading is not in the ideal zone.

Readings Below 6.5

At first, most people will have low pH readings due to the acid-forming tendency of the standard American diet. In this case, increase your intake of vegetables, fruits, root crops, nuts, seeds, and spices, striving to get 80% of your nutrition from these alkalizing foods. For details on the acid or alkaline-forming nature of various foods; see *The Acid-Alkaline Food Guide* (Square One Publishers, 2006).

Readings Above 7.5

A highly alkaline reading is likely due to catabolism, the process of breakdown of body tissue which triggers excess nitrogen in the urine. If you are consistently getting readings at 8.0, contact your health professional about how to stimulate the repair state to reverse this catabolic cycle.

Be patient and persistent. Remember, your pH indicates your reserve of alkaline minerals. It can take time to build up these reserves. Do not be discouraged with a slow movement towards the ideal alkaline measurement. It may have taken decades to get where you are; a few months to sustained repair and renewal are well worth the effort and attention.

Monitor Your pH Over Time

You do not have to measure your pH every day, but it is an excellent idea to keep some record of your pH test results over time. At the Center for Better Bones we use a Monthly pH Testing Record. You might want to use this chart yourself. As you incorporate our Alkaline for Life® Eating Program, and as you use supplements like ours which alkalize, you will see your pH reading move into the desired range.

Source: www.tinyurl.com/betterbones-alkalinebalance

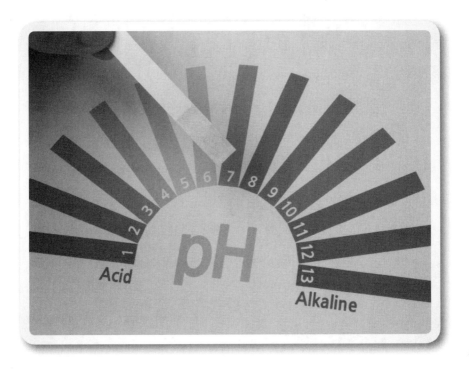

Almond Butter Squash

Pineapple **Lifestyle** Bay Leaf

Almond Milk Cabbage

Almonds Figs Flax seed **Sesame Seeds**

Apple Cider Vinegar Maca Chlorella Cacao Smoothies

Apples

Ginger

Gluten Free **Alkaline**

Superfoods NON GMO Lentils

RESIST
TEMPTATIONS

Kiwi Fruit **Spirulina**

Avocado **Strawberries**

Baking Soda Kidney Beans

Black Pepper **Grapes** **Hemp Hearts**

Blueberries **Himalayan Salt**

Kale **Brazil nuts**

Healing Green Tea **Acai**

Mango Lemons Green Juices

Garlic **Turmeric**

Tomatoes **Bok Choy**

Arugula **Sunflower Seeds**

28

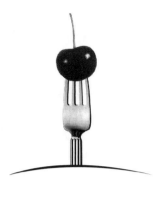

CHAPTER 4

Resisting The Temptations

Gluten

*O*nce you become a vegan you become aware of the incredible number of food items that are available to you.

While looking at food items in stores you notice now that most stores have a gluten-free section or many brands that are touting to be gluten free. This is a direct result of people who have adverse reactions to Gluten in foods. The most severe reaction to gluten is celiac disease.

Alarmingly, a majority of people have issues with gluten but don't know it or it shows as a symptom to another disease. So, in fact, a disease could be called cancer but is really rooted in gluten.

Gluten is a protein which originates from wheat but which is not metabolized by the body. Gluten is the cause of what is known as the *Wheat Belly,* a book made famous by Dr. William Davis.

As you start to truly look at labels, you start to see that wheat is in everything. Wheat intolerance is a scourge of the Western diet. Gluten is an allergen that is the root of many problems, including dry skin, irritability, eczema, and fatigue, to name a few, along with others in the video link below.

Excerpt below from Dr. Mark Hyman's
***Gluten: What You Don't Know Might Kill You*[2]**

Gluten Sensitivity: One Cause, Many Diseases

Something you're eating may be killing you, and you probably don't even know it! If you eat cheeseburgers or French fries all the time, or drink six sodas a day, you likely know you are shortening your life. But eating a nice dark, crunchy slice of whole wheat bread—how could that be bad for you? Well, bread contains gluten, a protein found in wheat, barley, rye, spelt, kamut, and oats. It is hidden in pizza, pasta, bread, wraps, rolls, and most processed foods. Clearly, gluten is a staple of the American diet. What most people don't know is that gluten can cause serious health complications for many. You may be at risk even if you don't have full-blown celiac disease. I want to reveal the truth about gluten, and explain the dangers.

And it's not just a few who suffer, but millions. Far more people have gluten sensitivity than you think—especially those

2   www.tinyurl.com/drhyman-what-you-dont-know

who are chronically ill. The most serious form of allergy to gluten, celiac disease, affects 1 in 100 people, or three million Americans, most of whom don't know they have it. But milder forms of gluten sensitivity are even more common and may affect up to one-third of the American population.

Something you're eating may be killing you, and you probably don't even know it!

Why haven't you heard much about this?

Well, actually you have, but you just don't realize it. Celiac disease and gluten sensitivity masquerade as dozens and dozens of other diseases with different names.

A review paper in the *New England Journal of Medicine* listed 55 "diseases" that can be caused by eating gluten. These include osteoporosis, irritable bowel disease, inflammatory bowel disease, anemia, cancer, fatigue, canker sores, (v) and rheumatoid arthritis, lupus, multiple sclerosis, and almost all other autoimmune diseases. Gluten is also linked to many psychiatric and neurological diseases, including anxiety, depression, schizophrenia, dementia, migraines, epilepsy, and neuropathy (nerve damage). It has also been linked to autism.

Gluten sensitivity is actually an autoimmune disease that creates inflammation throughout the body, with wide-ranging effects across all organ systems including your brain, heart, joints, digestive tract, and more. It can be the single cause behind many different "diseases." To correct these diseases, you need to treat the cause—which is often gluten sensitivity—not just the symptoms.

Of course, that doesn't mean that ALL cases of depression or autoimmune disease or any of these other problems are caused by gluten in everyone—but it is important to look for it if you have any chronic illnesses.

The question that remains is: Why are we so sensitive to this "staff of life," the staple of our diet?

There are many reasons …

They include our lack of genetic adaptation to grasses, and particularly gluten, in our diet. Wheat was introduced into Europe during the Middle Ages, and thirty percent of people of European descent carry the gene for celiac disease (HLA DQ2 or HLA DQ8), (xii) which increases susceptibility to health problems from eating gluten.

American strains of wheat have a much higher gluten content (which is needed to make light, fluffy Wonder Bread and giant bagels) than those traditionally found in Europe. This super-gluten was recently introduced into our agricultural food supply and now has "infected" nearly all wheat strains in America.

To find out if you are one of the millions of people suffering from an unidentified gluten sensitivity, just follow this simple procedure:

The Elimination/Reintegration Diet

While testing can help identify gluten sensitivity, the only way you will know if this is really a problem for you is to eliminate all gluten for a short period of time (two to four weeks) and see how you feel. Get rid of the following foods:

- Gluten (barley, rye, oats, spelt, kamut, wheat, triticale—see www.celiac.com for a complete list of foods that contain gluten, as well as often surprising and hidden sources of gluten)

- Hidden sources (soup mixes, salad dressings, sauces, as well as lipstick, certain vitamins, medications, stamps, and envelopes you have to lick, and even Play-Doh)

For this test to work you MUST eliminate 100 percent of the gluten from your diet—no exceptions. No hidden gluten, and not a single crumb of bread.

So one of the main keys to amazing health is to eliminate gluten completely and permanently from our bodies, our kitchen, and our lifestyle. No exceptions. No cheating. This is an empowerment point, and your body will reward you quickly with a little extra weight loss and added energy, as it did for me.

> **So one of the main keys to amazing health is to eliminate gluten completely and permanently from our bodies, our kitchen, and our lifestyle. No exceptions. No cheating.**

Once you have actively removed gluten from your diet, and then add it back in with a piece of toast or bun, you will notice the difference in how your body responds and how you feel.

As Dr. Mark Hyman mentions, you can't have crumb of gluten. This means that if you order a salad without croutons and it arrives with croutons, you don't just pick them out. Nor do you send back the salad for the kitchen to pick them out. You must get a whole new salad or change your order, because they won't make a new salad; they will simply just pull out the croutons and your salad is tainted. It only takes a few crumbs to pollute your body with gluten.

It is to be noted that the centenarians[3] of the world, the people who have lived the longest, have for many years, if not their whole lives, not been exposed to gluten, e.g., the Okinawans of Japan, who have one of the highest populations of centenarians in the world.

So now that you have eliminated animal products and animal by-products such as cheese, milk, yogurt, cream, and butter, you've laid the foundation of the vegan lifestyle. You can work towards an alkaline body. To supercharge this process, eliminate gluten if you haven't already.

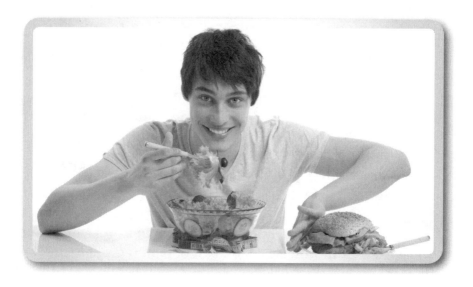

3   www.genarians.com

Eliminating gluten is to avoid wheat flour, oats, kamut, and rye, but mostly you will see wheat flour in some percentage or another in many foods on the shelves today. That will include products like ketchup, soya sauce, frozen dinners, all bread (unless otherwise stated gluten free) and beer (beer belly/wheat belly).

Now that you've made these adjustments in your food intake and awareness of food purchases, you've come a long way. Congratulations!

This change of diet, in combination with a daily exercise protocol of at least twenty minutes of cardio exercise, has already shown you many benefits and built confidence. Now with the elimination of gluten, you will start to see and resonate with new levels of energy. As such, now would be a good time to start improving your cardiovascular exercise routine to a higher standard.

I know some people love their beer, but beer has to go. You can't drink beer and think you're going to eliminate gluten. In fact, it's interesting to watch the advertising connection that beer companies have with exercise. They celebrate athletic achievement with the drinking of beer. Yet beer contains gluten; even light beer contains gluten, and gluten has a direct co-relation to ill health and auto-immune diseases, as proven by the current research available.

Now that you have this information, you understand why in most supermarkets gluten-free is an emerging section dedicated to gluten-free products. The market is demanding this troublesome protein to be removed from our foods as often it's used as filled, and as being a direct source to disease. The consumer demand is proof that a growing section of society knows of the perils, and is driving more people towards a vegetarian and vegan lifestyle as no gluten exists in plants, only in wheat, kamut, oats, rye and barley, but not in lemons, kale, carrots, Swiss chard, and beets. It's only in grains.

There are many good gluten-free products available in today's food stores, including gluten-free rice tortillas, many GF breads, GF potato chips, gluten-free tamari, GF this and GF that—the list is ever growing.

Gluten-free is an important key in maintaining amazing health. For myself, I lost additional weight once I went gluten-free. Weight dropped, skin cleaned up. Now note this is a process, because until you start, you don't know where wheat is hiding. But by now you've become a good label reader. If by accident you purchase something with gluten, take it back. I do, and I tell them why.

In fact, the more you buy gluten-free, the more the retailers will stock gluten-free items to satisfy the demand. Take control; be part of the food revolution for you and for others.

I think it's important to mention to chart what you're doing so you can see your workouts, your weight loss, your food purchases, and your money savings/costs, so you have a rough idea of your incredible journey to amazing health.

> **Take control; be part of the food revolution for you and for others.**

Now we're getting somewhere!!! You're really on track now. You've joined the next level: VEGAN PLUS. Give yourself a high five. ☺

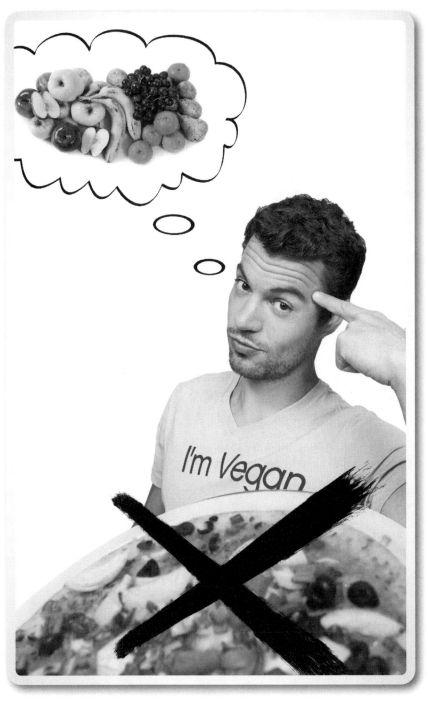

Spirulina
Avocado Strawberries
Baking Soda
Black Pepper Kidney Beans
Grapes Hemp Hearts
Blueberries Himalayan Salt
Kale Brazil nuts
Healing Green Tea
Mango Lemons Green Juices
Garlic Turmeric
Tomatoes Bok Choy
Arugula Sunflower Seeds
SUGAR Acai
Almond Butter Kiwi Fruit
Squash
Pineapple Lifestyle
Almond Milk Cabbage Bay Leaf
Almonds Figs Flax seed Sesame Seeds
Apple Cider Vinegar Maca Chlorella Cacao Smoothies
Apples
Ginger
Gluten Free Alkaline
Superfoods NON GMO Lentils

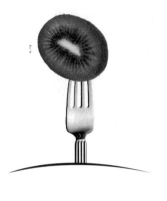

CHAPTER 5

Sugar

*A*s far as back as most of us can remember, sugar has been a part of our lives as a treat. We are given candy, sweets and celebrations, birthday parties require cake; you went to the fair, you got candy floss; trick-or-treating at Halloween is all about receiving candy, more sugar! As young adults, a lot of emphasis is put on soda pop, ice cream, donuts, and eventually, you come of age and now alcohol is available to you. Alcohol is sugar. Many diners still offer cubes of sugar in bowls on their tables for coffee.

"When you eat sugar, a process known as glycation occurs. The sugar in your bloodstream attaches to proteins to form harmful new molecules called 'advanced glycation end products,' which then damage adjacent proteins, such as collagen and elastin, as well as increasing the risk of age-related diseases such as cataracts, Alzheimer's disease, heart disease and stroke. Additionally, a diet

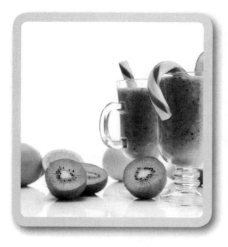

high in sugar will actually cause the body to create less resilient new collagen! So even a young person on a high-sugar diet is setting himself or herself up for premature aging. But not all is lost! Cutting sugar from your diet can allow your body to repair the damage and rebuild weakened collagen." (Excerpt from *One Green Planet*, October 5, 2014)

Two modern-day tragedies of epidemic proportions have risen in our modern era, and they are called diabetes and obesity.

The liver cannot process sugar, so the liver turns it into fat. You end up with a fatty liver. The pancreas maintains the body's blood sugar levels by producing insulin when there is too much sugar in the blood, thereby creating an imbalance which triggers diabetes. The harmony of the body is disrupted by sugar.

Sugar is in almost all food you eat. However, there is enough glucose in plants, fruits, and vegetables in a natural state that satisfy and maintain the blood sugar balance. Today our society provides food with excessive amounts in everything you eat. Anything processed is loaded with sugar. Interesting point is that to eat the so-called "low fat" means high sugar replacing the fat.

> **Interesting point is that to eat the so-called "low fat" means high sugar replacing the fat.**

Because of the diabetes epidemic, artificial sweeteners often replace real sugar in an attempt to reduce the diabetic problem. Soda pops are no longer sweetened by cane sugar, but more by lab-created artificial sweeteners. Names like aspartame, NutraSweet, fructose, and maltodextrin, for example, are names you may know.

> **Excerpt from Dr. Joseph Mercola**
>
> - A 2009 study from the University of California[4], Davis shows how a high-fructose diet can cause you to build new fat cells around your heart, liver, and digestive organs in just 10 weeks, plunging you into the early stages of diabetes and heart disease (whereas a high glucose diet did not have the same effects).
> - Excess fructose consumption is a major contributor to insulin resistance and obesity, hypertension, cardiovascular disease, liver disease, cancer, arthritis, and other diseases.
> - Fructose is metabolized very differently in your body from glucose; all of the metabolic burden falls on your liver, in much the same way as for alcohol, and your body becomes a sea of toxic by-products.
> - Glucose, on the other hand, is your body's nearly ideal source of fuel, meaning it has none of the damaging metabolic effects of fructose; glucose also suppresses your appetite, unlike fructose, which stimulates your appetite and encourages overeating and the accumulation of excess body fat.

Sugar suppresses the immune system and plays havoc with your pancreas, causing your body to go out of balance and attacking your system.

---

4   articles.mercola.com/sites/articles/archive/2010/01/02/highfructose-corn-syrup-alters-human-metabolism.aspx

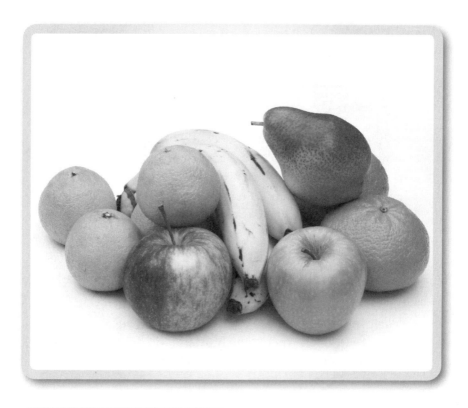

The good sugar you are looking for is in an apple, banana, dates, figs, and oranges, all excellent substitutes instead of reaching for refined sugar.

Most of us know that feeling that we want something sweet, and we go to great lengths to get it. Perhaps it's candy, donuts, coffee; it's sitting at every counter at every store around. The good sugar you are looking for is in an apple, banana, dates, figs, and oranges, all excellent substitutes instead of reaching for refined sugar.

Excerpt from Dr. Sanjay Gupta

Source: www.everydayhealth.com/sanjay-gupta/myths-and-facts-about-sugar-substitutes.aspx

"Sugar substitutes are much sweeter than sugar, which can have an adverse effect on how we choose what foods to eat. If you're having a lot of artificial sweeteners, they can increase your preference for them and make more nutritious foods less tasty and appealing," said Alexandra Kaplan Corwin, a registered dietician in the division of pediatric endocrinology and diabetes at The Children's Hospital at Montefiore Medical Center in New York City.

Here's how 5 FDA-approved artificial sweeteners measure up on the "sweetness scale," according to the Sugar Association:

- Acesulfame Potassium[5], or Ace-K, is 200 times sweeter than sugar.
- Aspartame (marketed as Equal and NutraSweet) is 200 times sweeter than sugar.
- Neotame is about 40 times sweeter than aspartame, or 8,000 times sweeter than sugar.
- Saccharine (commonly sold as Sweet 'N Low) can be between 200 and 700 times sweeter than sugar.
- Sucralose (sold as Splenda) is 600 times sweeter than sugar.

Here are some healthy tips on consuming sugar and sugar substitutes:

- If you're looking to avoid both sugary and artificially sweetened drinks, try water or seltzer flavored with fruit slices or mint leaves.

5   www.tinyurl.com/what-is-acesulfame-potassium

- Among sugar substitutes, Corwin prefers the natural sweetener stevia, which is derived from a plant. Refined stevia extract is generally regarded as safe, but the FDA hasn't approved it in whole-leaf or crude form because of concerns about possible side-effects.

- When buying juice drinks for your kids, look for the phrase "100 percent juice." Those juices will contain the vitamins and minerals found in the fruit, said King. Avoid products that are "fruit flavored."

Sugar destroys your health, and as Dr. Sanjay Gupta expresses in the link above, sugar is now becoming known as a toxin. The amount that is now being consumed per person per day is reaching toxic levels, in all of us eating a Western diet in particular. Sugar is in at least 80% of products offered on the shelf and in restaurant food you order.

Easily I can say that in my lifetime of 57 years, compared to my teenage daughter of eighteen years, the difference in the health of the children from when I grew up to her generation is frightening. I am blessed to have grown up prior to the fast-food industry arriving. When I was young, I had never heard of the diseases we all know of today. I think there was one person in my high school who had diabetes, but it wasn't an epidemic. That has changed. Prior to the fast-food industry arriving, food was more home-prepared and costly, so the "treats" of sugar were few and far between. Sugar and sweets were something we looked forward to, not expected every day. We naturally ate fruits and veggies because that's what was served on millions of tables in homes throughout the '50s, '60s, and '70s, with only tiny portions of meat. Meat portions have grown to four or five times the portions of the veggies, with sometimes no veggies at all. You get a massive steak with a baked potato and a tiny broccoli spear. The serving portions were opposite when I was growing up and people were thin, including our parents.

High fructose corn syrup is replacing refined white sugar because corn subsidies have helped make this sweetener cheap and very widespread. High fructose corn syrup is also fed to animals in feed lots and is being used in soda pops and boxed, processed foods, including cereals, gum, candies, and cakes; anything you can consider to be sweet has some form of artificial sweetener.

For example, according to *Time Magazine* (June 23, 2014), since 1970 the calories in soda pop have risen 8,853% with the inclusion of high fructose corn syrup. This is, of course, a horrifying leap that is creating an epidemic.

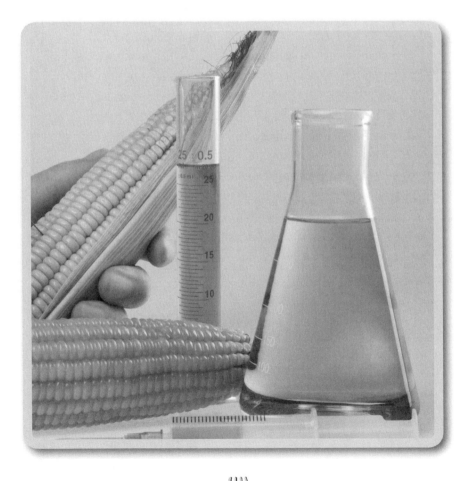

Excerpt from Wikipedia on *King Corn*

Early on in the vegan journey we came across a great film called *King Corn*[6]. *King Corn* is a 2007 documentary film released in October 2007 following college friends Ian Cheney and Curtis Ellis (directed by Aaron Woolf) as they move from Boston to Greene, Iowa to grow and farm an acre of corn. In the process, Cheney and Ellis examine the role that the increasing production of corn has had for American society, spotlighting the role of government subsidies in encouraging the huge amount of corn grown.

The film shows how industrialization in corn has all but eliminated the image of the family farm, which is being replaced by larger industrial farms. Cheney and Ellis suggest that this trend reflects a larger industrialization of the North American food system. As was outlined in the film, decisions relating to what crops are grown and how they are grown are based on government manipulated economic considerations rather than their true economic, environmental, or social ramifications. This is demonstrated in the film by the production of high fructose corn syrup, an ingredient found in many cheap food products, such as fast-food.

One of the first things we did in our experience was eliminate bread right away because of the sugar and the gluten. Bread is mostly not good for you. I haven't missed bread at all. You have to put things on it so you need butter, jam, peanut butter, margarine, jellies, vegemite, or preserves, and all of these things are filled with sugar.

6   www.tinyurl.com/wiki-Kingcorn

So we replaced bread with gluten-free brown rice tortillas, which we still use today in wraps, pizza bases, or you can cut into squares for dips with hummus, or you can dip in soups so it's like your little croutons.

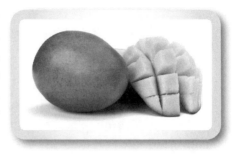

In our third year of being vegan, we finally got to a place where we let go of alcohol, because alcohol is sugar. It converts to sugar—it is sugar. Wine, beers, spirits—all the popular alcohol marketed to young people that's pre-mixed, mixes—it's all sugar, and this is part of the epidemic.

Our children have already had childhood and adolescent years of ingesting a lot of toxins. If parents aren't taking care of what the children are eating, then soda pop and candy bars are the tip of the sugar disaster awaiting them. The fast-food industry offers an alarming array of sugar in their meals, hidden everywhere, from the meat to the drinks, to fries to the ice creams. These are sugar stores, as liquor is a sugar store.

Letting go of alcohol is an important health step. Many celebrations and parties revolve around alcohol as a social aspect of the gathering. By eliminating all alcohol I instantly lost another five pounds and more. Suddenly I could run further and faster; instantly I had more energy, less weight, better skin, and overall, a better feeling of well-being. It was during a time when I was serving wine that I discovered that animal products are used in wine making!! What??? This information fortified my decision to stop taking alcohol, as it is not part of a healthy lifestyle.

Excerpt from *Time Magazine*, June 23, 2014

"It can be hard to understand why a diet heavy in refined carbs can lead to obesity and diabetes. It has to do with blood chemistry. Simple carbs like bread and corn may not look like sugar on your plate, but in your body, that's what they're converted to when digested." (Page 34 by Bryan Walsh.)

"Dr. Dariush Mozaffarian, the incoming Dean of Nutrition Science at Tufts University, says 'a bagel is no different than a bag of Skittles in your body.'"

In summary, even baked goods now cannot be part of a Vegan Plus Diet. Flour (gluten), butter (animal product), sugar (toxin), and eggs (animal product), along with a long list of chemicals, cannot be considered a key for amazing health. You must get away from packaged foods and move to plants, and mostly raw.

A few excellent sweeteners I have found and use are dates, figs, fruits such as bananas, and if you have to you could use stevia (although I never have), which shows the most promise from a plant.

Read your labels, and anything labeled that you don't know what it is, you must put back on the shelf. You don't need sweeteners really; it's mind over matter. You don't need to satisfy something for a moment of satisfaction for a lifetime of mounting health problems. I have been part of the sugar addiction. I have eaten bowls full of ice cream, several in a sitting. Sugar is a serious problem that you must address from a position that you can control it and it is easy, but first you must eliminate it as a process so that eventually, you get to almost none.

> **Don't be fooled by labels and green-washing.**

As a footnote, these days, if I purchase something and find it has toxic ingredients I take it back, even if opened. I continuously educate myself about the dangers of that food, and I take that to the grocer so that he/she knows, and perhaps they won't sell it anymore. Remember, your vote counts at the till.

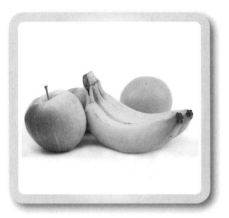

Don't be fooled by labels and green-washing.

I have been through enough to know that you can be easily tricked at the store, and by the pressures of society and the marketing around these "products." Recently, for example, I purchased an Aloe Vera drink, and I didn't read the label for some reason. I am not a robot. It's a plant-based drink that is sold in stores with a good reputation. When I took a sip, I knew it had something very sweet and sure enough, it was high fructose corn syrup. I was shocked! I took it back! I got a full refund, and explained the dangers to the shop owner, who was not at all aware of the perils of high fructose corn syrup.

> **What he does with his store is not my business, but where I shop and what I purchase and put in my body is my business.**

What he does with his store is not my business, but where I shop and what I purchase and put in my body is my business.

Get involved with the business of your health. If I can make these changes, you can make these changes. It's a matter of how much you want the results of gaining back your health.

Avocado
Spirulina
Strawberries
Baking Soda
Black Pepper
Kidney Beans
Grapes
Hemp Hearts
Blueberries
Himalayan Salt
Acai
Kale
Brazil nuts
DISCPLINE
Healing
Green Tea
Mango
Lemons
Green Juices
Garlic
Turmeric
Tomatoes
Bok Choy
Arugula
Sunflower Seeds
Kiwi Fruit
Almond Butter
Squash
Pineapple
Lifestyle
Almond Milk
Cabbage
Bay Leaf
Almonds
Figs
Flax seed
Sesame Seeds
Apple Cider Vinegar
Apples
Maca
Chlorella
Cacao
Smoothies
Ginger
Alkaline
Gluten Free
Superfoods
NON GMO
Lentils

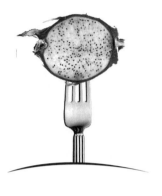

C H A P T E R   6

Sustaining Vegan Discipline Ethical Choices

*S*ustaining your newfound vegan lifestyle may seem
challenging for a number of reasons. These challenges may
include: Negative feedback from friends and family, difficulty of
detaching from ingrained habits (sugar, processed foods, fast-foods,
animal products, beliefs, etc.) and discipline.

In this chapter I will discuss and touch upon some of these
points to help you overcome or understand where some of your
challenges may come from.

Sustaining vegan is a wonderful discipline. It's kind of like
quitting smoking, if you've ever done it. It's highly beneficial to your

> **Sustaining vegan is a wonderful discipline.**

longevity of life. As an example, you've learned the benefits of going through the changes when you quit smoking, lose weight, start exercising. You start to see the benefits.

It starts with discipline and ends up with a lifestyle you couldn't have expected, but which you enjoy so much once you start.

All disciplines have rising temptations to derail your resolve and try to undermine your ability to stay the course.

There are two types of influences: internal and external. Both are powerful because they are equally run by the ego, and are entrenched in society as being the way you should live. This has been happening to us since our birth.

Sustaining vegan opens new doors for our wellness that even those of us who think we are well—and I was one of those people—are not, until we make a quantum shift and stick with it.

By internal influences I mean triggers such as an odor. As we all know, the smell of a flower can bring you back to childhood. The smell of a perfume can bring you back to a date. The same as the odor of a steak house, a coffee shop perhaps, a bakery, a fast-food place, can take you back to memories or feelings associated with that. Now you have taken the leap to follow the discipline of your newfound lifestyle, motivated by your growing, ever so healthy results.

Staying the course and going through the challenges with your newfound knowledge, desires, and successes fortifies your willpower to keep to your newfound discipline and maintain the vegan lifestyle.

"Don't bend back—lean forward."

—SUZANNE MILES

Discipline is okay. It's powerful. Discipline is something you build; it's not special or specific to any one person. It's available for everyone. It's critical to your long-term success.

I have found that the longer I stay with the vegan lifestyle and the discipline, at the time of this writing (three years, four months), the more I learn, the more I grow, the more I glow. ☺

The benefits are in the long haul.

The benefits are in everything you have overcome.

Which leads me to external influences: We are heavily influenced on many levels externally. Some examples are annual celebrations, such as Thanksgiving, Christmas, and Easter. Then social gatherings such as barbeques, birthday parties, dinner dates, picnics. Then there is the marketing on how you should be, what you should eat, and the events you must shop for and attend as seen on media such as TV, radio, Facebook, billboards, media advertising, and the news.

> **Discipline is something you build; it's not special or specific to any one person. It's available for everyone. It's critical to your long-term success.**

These are the times that test your resolve. You can use these as opportunities to flex your ever more strengthening willpower. Which is easy. Your plant-based lifestyle is giving you many more benefits and results than the other way ever did.

As people have no idea of the strength of your discipline, they will want to tempt your resolve. This is mostly friends and family.

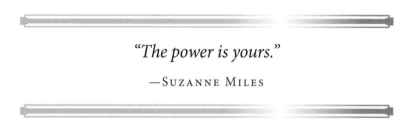

"The power is yours."

—SUZANNE MILES

People will want to test your discipline with temptations, especially on festive gathering occasions. For example, at a birthday party: "Come on, Suzanne, have a piece of cake. I made it myself. It won't hurt you. It's your dad's birthday! Come on."

They have no idea of the strength of my resolve now. It's such a powerful position built on the knowledge that my previous lifestyle led me to an unhealthy, premature aging, being overweight, following the system in a sick condition. That is motivational resolve unto itself. It is the foundation of the stories you see about someone losing 120 pounds, for example, or an athlete who rises to the top, or an entrepreneurial rags-to-riches story. This is discipline working for you!

Anyone can change even me, starting all over again at age 54. You can lose weight; you can bring your cholesterol back to normal levels without medication. Medication has a place, but mostly it's a business.

However, there is another resolve to consider that factors into your willpower. ETHICAL CHOICES. Ethical choices naturally develop the longer you stay true to the vegan lifestyle. Everyone starts for different reasons—for some it's weight loss and body image, for others it's love of animals; for another they're sick and tired of being sick and tired. For others it's a show or a documentary they saw about feedlots and antibiotics in animals; for others it's animal treatment and abuse. Some people suddenly wake up and don't want the industrial system to feed them anymore.

I would like to make a point here that many children are interested in vegetarian[7] options, and I think they are to be taken seriously with this request and supported.

Six suggested resources to gain information about the industrial manufacturing of food:

- ***King Corn*** – "*King Corn* is a feature documentary about two friends, one acre of corn, and the subsidized crop that drives our fast-food nation. In *King Corn*, Ian Cheney and Curt Ellis, best friends from college on the East Coast, move to the heartland to learn where their food comes from. With the help of friendly neighbors, genetically modified seeds, and powerful herbicides, they plant and grow a bumper crop of America's most-productive, most-subsidized grain on one acre of Iowa soil. But when they try to follow their pile of corn into the food system, what they find raises troubling questions about how we eat—and how we farm."–*Written by King Corn* www.imdb.com/title/tt1112115

---

7   www.youtube.com/watch?v=sJNntUXyWvw

55

- *Food Inc.* – An unflattering look inside America's corporately controlled food industry. imdb.com/title/tt1286537

- *Our Daily Bread* "is a wide-screen tableau of a feast which isn't always easy to digest—and in which we all take part. A pure, meticulous and high-end film experience that enables the audience to form their own ideas." www.youtube.com/watch?v=pVkieJ_Wj64

- *Earthlings* – Using hidden cameras and never-before-seen footage, *EARTHLINGS* chronicles the day-to-day practices of the largest industries in the world, all of which rely entirely on animals for profit. www.earthlings.com

- *Forks Over Knives* – Warning, this movie could save your life. www.forksoverknives.com

- *Sweet Revenge: Turning The Table on Processed Food* – *Dr. Robert H. Lustig*

> **There is a vegan movement going on and it's growing. This is a great time to be part of a wonderful change in the taking back of our food.**

There is much astonishing and often shocking information to reflect on from these sources. These are just a few of a plethora out there. You likely will look at food differently after seeing these. I did. My husband and children did, as have millions of others around the world.

There is a vegan movement going on and it's growing. This is a great time to be part of a wonderful change in the taking back of our food.

When you watch these films, you get an understanding of how the animals are treated and how they are fed. You realize that your ethical choice to not have any part of that process becomes an easy one. In fact, it is as Ellen DeGeneres says in her interview[8] with Katy Couric.

> *"I just had a disconnect. I decided it was more important for me to taste a cheeseburger and have a steak or a turkey sandwich and it's just easier. I just put it out of mind."*
>
> —ELLEN DEGENERES

For me personally, I have on occasions fed a cow with a handful of grass and petted the cow's forehead and looked into its eyes, and never once in that great moment of connection to a rather large, docile animal did I consider to eat any part of its flesh or organs, or use its skin for my purpose. This is the connection. The food system disconnects and turns their bodies into marketing pieces called food.

My family and I have learned this, because we, too, never thought about this connection when we ate food from the "industrial system." If we had to slaughter, skin, gut, and prepare any part of the animal for ourselves, we wouldn't be able to do it. The enjoyment of picking greens, vegetables, fruits, nuts, beans, herbs, and spices is so much easier and clean, from preparation to clean up, and so much healthier for your body, mind, and spirit. We really do have an ethical decision that fortifies our food choices. We are no longer contributing to animal cruelty.

8   www.youtube.com/watch?v=UeSA2j4oiDA&feature=youtu.be

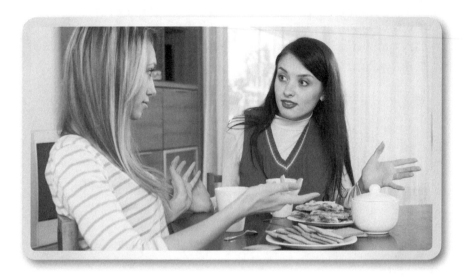

When one combines an ethical choice with a motivational, result-driven, plant-based lifestyle, the two work in synergy to fortify your willpower to stay true to yourself and your goals. It doesn't matter what others think.

The willpower to stay the course becomes stronger and unyielding as you continue to learn, grow and develop an amazing new lifestyle. Healthy eating habits and healthy exercise efforts guide you towards a healthy you, in body, mind and spirit. You feel better. You are more in control. Your curiosity will continue to grow, and you continually are in a process of eliminating the industrial food systems status quo that threatens your health.

Ethical choices are at the checkout. Your vote is at the checkout. You vote with everything you buy.

An ethical choice isn't just about animals; it also about chemical additives, herbicides, pesticides, and antibiotics that are introduced without our knowledge into everyday foods by the industrial food machine. There is a toxic chemical slurry of food additives going into everyday foods, mostly packaged and processed. With the rise of epidemics of obesity, type 2 diabetes, heart disease, cancer, Alzheimer's, gallstones, skin disorders, mental health issues, ADHD, and many more, could there be a correlation between the food we are given in stores to this surge of dis-eases amongst our modern society? I say yes because I, too, was a victim. If you don't know what the label means you shouldn't buy it. Period!

Organic foods, or growing your own, is the best you can have. Spend your money wisely on these food choices. The ethical choices of buying no animal products and choosing pesticide-free, chemical-free, organically grown (preferably by small farms) fruits and vegetables is currently having a positive growth surge in our stores.

The advent of organic sections in supermarkets is proof that a growing segment of the public is becoming much more aware, and is requesting and choosing organic and gluten-free foods for their health.

Vegetarians and vegans enjoy impressive, well-documented health advantages. There are many recognized examples of people recovering from illness and disease through pure, clean, plant-based food. One of the optimal gifts of this lifestyle is greater longevity and happiness. Not being sick because of your age is a critical point of freedom. Not having age-related illnesses, and being able to ward off disease offers a wonderful sense of self-realization, empowerment, and motivation. Why would we accept diseases such as cancer, obesity, cataracts, and gallstones as part of our life?

Being vegetarian and vegan does not guarantee a healthy body. After all, potato chips, cola, and many other fatty, salty and sugary foods are called vegetarian/vegan but are not good for you. Beware of green-washing and mass-produced "vegan food." Vegan food can be laden with sugar, salt, sweeteners, hidden chemicals, and be harmful for you, too. It is important to know the difference between living a vegan lifestyle and being a consumer. For example, I'm not going down the aisle looking for vegan ice cream. I know it's there, but I'm sticking to the discipline of the plants. That's where the wellness is.

This is a key!

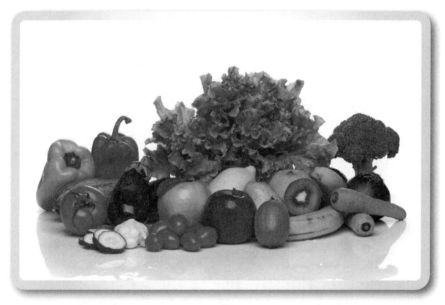

The highest rates of longevity in the world are in areas where vegetables, legumes, nuts, fruits, seeds, and spices are the dominant food staples. These foods offer many protectors of disease to the body and are readily available, and are part of those peoples' wisdom of food for body, mind, and spirit.

The challenges to sustain vegan are common to all who make this transition, especially in Western society. However, there are many ways to and advantages of overcoming these challenges, as discussed here.

Welcome, and be proud of being part of the new food revolution, taking back your health, enjoying spending your money ethically on good food that serves your body, mind, and spirit, and gives you the best chance for a healthy, lengthy life. This is your time. Enjoy it!

This is your time. Enjoy it!

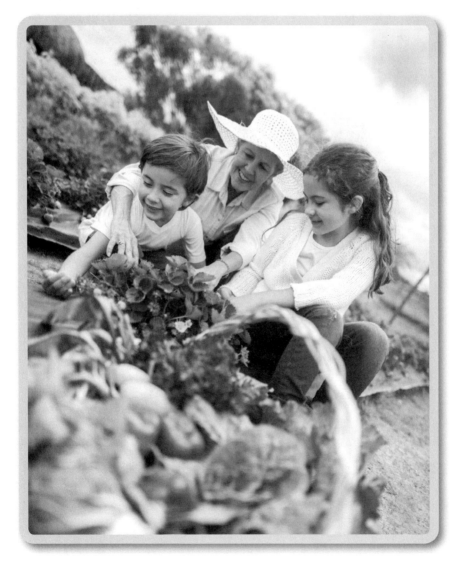

Almond Butter

Kiwi Fruit

Squash

Pineapple

Lifestyle

Almond Milk Cabbage

Bay Leaf

Almonds Figs

Flax seed Sesame Seeds

Apple Cider Vinegar Maca

Smoothies

Apples Chlorella Cacao

Acai Spirulina Kale Brazil nuts

Gluten Free Healing Strawberries

GMO

Blueberries

Ginger

Grapes

Green Tea

Mango Lemons Green Juices

Garlic Turmeric

Tomatoes Bok Choy

Arugula Sunflower Seeds

Superfoods NON GMO Lentils

Kidney Beans

Hemp Hearts

Baking Soda Black Pepper Himalayan Salt

Avocado Alkaline

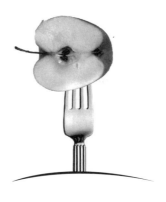

CHAPTER 7

Genetically Modified Foods (GMO) And The Reasons To Support Local, Independent, And Small Farmers

*I*t is an interesting fact that our food gets tampered with and changed without any input or consent from the population of consumers. What I have discovered, and was involved in prior to embracing the plant-based lifestyle, was a "system" that I was disconnected from, although I thought I was knowledgeable about my purchasing and what I ate.

New methods of high-yield farming are employed. Artificial foods and flavors are created in a lab and added to food. Yet you and

I, the consumer, are not informed of the dangers of this chemical slurry unless we read labels and know what they mean.

Genetically modified foods, otherwise known as GMO, are a hot topic of discussion, with many people around the world demanding more information and labeling of such foods. Groups such as the Non-GMO Project[9] are very active in informing people of the hazards of GMO in their food.

Look for packaged foods, if you must buy them at all, bearing the Non-GMO Project label. You will find it on items like potato chips, breads and tamari sauce.

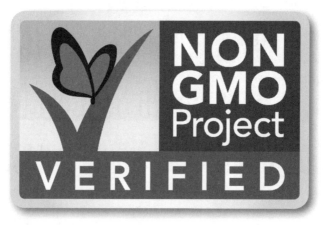

It is widely accepted that if a food item is for sale in a food store that it is safe to eat. We have this wired misconception of programming that the food in the store must be safe, otherwise why would it be there? This we now know to be false because of the burgeoning health crisis of many populations around the world, including obesity, heart disease, cancer, diabetes, mental health issues, autoimmune diseases, ADHD, and many other health problems that have risen to a global epidemic.

---

9   www.nongmoproject.org

My first-hand knowledge that I was a victim of this unsafe food was my awakening at 54 years of age that I really was pretty much obese. I had high cholesterol. I had premature aging, I had a massive fibroid, and was looking at major surgery. I was sent to the Healthy Heart Clinic for testing and involvement in their program. I wasn't even 50 years old then! There I found myself with all these other people with similar health problems. Some people had heart attacks and they weren't old, either. It wasn't until years later that I learned for myself that at the foundation of this crisis is food. The proof of that is that now my body has changed to amazing health and energy, an entirely new vibration.

The laneway of ill health was not going to be my story, and in the summer of 2011, I dug in and changed direction with a plant-based lifestyle. I told the surgeon that her story of what she was going to do to the long-term outcome and me was not my story, and I walked away! *Disclaimer* always check with your doctor and do your own research.

Industrial food developers, chemists, and lab technicians continue to tamper with food, searching for longer shelf life, flavors, binding agents, textures, and colors, even entirely new products that are made in a lab. They are busy "developing" food for the masses, not food for health.

Learning more about GMO foods quickly came into vision. This was an area I knew was out there but was disconnected from the actual extent of how powerful and deep GMO has gone into the food system in North America.

The GMO process is employed at the cellular level of seeds to increase crop yield by the bushel. For example, in the documentary *King Corn*, we learned that the crop yield of a GMO corn seed was 200 bushels per acre, and a non-GMO seed was 20 bushels per acre. We also learned that the cobs of the GMO seed were not edible and the farmers don't grow it to eat on their tables; it's grown for feeding cattle in feedlots and used as fillers for many foods in the supermarket.

The rest of the corn plant, including stems and leaves, are used to create high fructose corn syrup (HFCS) according to the *King Corn* documentary.[10]

High fructose corn syrup is a calorie-providing sweetener, which has a long list of unhealthy effects to our bodies, along with a growing variety of food products that use high fructose corn syrup as an ingredient. High fructose corn syrup comes from GMO corn. You cannot go into a field and squeeze HFCS from the plant; it has to be processed or manufactured and it's in all the beef, chicken and pork you eat en masse.

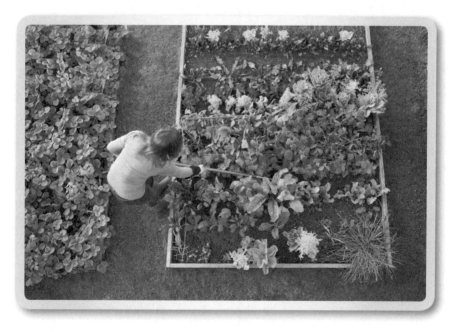

---

10   www.imdb.com/title/tt1112115

Excerpt from Dr. Joseph Mercola

"BAD TO THE LAST DROP: Refiners Squeeze Dangerous Additives From Corn"[11] is to tell you about high-fructose corn syrup, which has varied dangers that stare us in the face but still finds its way in foods, including:

- Baked goods
- Canned fruits
- Dairy products
- Carbonated drinks
- And most sweetened beverages in the market today

The creation of GMO foods and products, including those containing high fructose corn syrup, is another industrialized food manipulation that we learned to avoid in our plant-based lifestyle. There is much to learn about GMO foods and the power of their yield on the unsuspecting public. Just Google it and do your research. I'm sure you'll learn very quickly to get this out of your diet completely.

One of the best ways that I know of to avoid purchasing GMO produce and food is to find and support your local farmers and farmers markets. You can usually speak directly with the farmer. You can ask them about their product, and if it is GMO or not. You can ask about the soil and how they grow the food they are selling. You can find out a lot by directly speaking with these people. You may inspire a farmer to find new foods to grow for you. There are many supportive, interesting farmers ready to sell you good food.

---

11   www.tinyurl.com/ebook-highfructose-corn

It's a lot of fun to drive the 100-mile radius around where you live and find foods that are suitable for you. You also get a chance to reconnect with where your food is coming from. It educates you, so you are more powerful with your vote at the checkout and with a newfound informed ability to shop more wisely for you and your family.

Most likely there are stores in your town or nearby that are committed to selling only pesticide-free, chemical-free, GMO-free organically grown foods. The support you give to these often hardworking store owners gives the green light signal to the farmers to grow more, as you are now part of the new food revolution seeking better choices for the health of yourself and your family.

Locally, in my town, I have come to know several small businesses that seek and support organic farmers and suppliers. One is a small store called Tama Organic[12]. I love going to this store because they now know me by name. I can speak directly to the owner about the products. I often get free samples to try, and they are genuinely happy to see me. They take the time to show me new produce that has come in, and they know the benefits because they eat it themselves. They stay after hours if I phone them and let them know I am on my way—that's good customer service in my book!

When I ventured deeper into shopping for our food, it was evident that a new style of shopping was emerging. Sweet Cherubim[13] on Commercial Drive in Vancouver is a long-standing vegetarian/vegan restaurant and supermarket offering a wide array of healthy and interesting products for the healthy consumer. The general manager, Brig Chopra, wishes that everybody would become at least vegetarian, if not vegan, for their health and that of the planet.

---

12   www.tamaorganic.com

13   www.sweetcherubim.com

It was in these stores that I learned so much more about food, as the store owners themselves have educational information and genuinely care about the products they sell. An example of that is garlic. There is a big difference between beautiful, plump, organic garlic bulbs oozing with the healthy allicin oils under the skin and covered in dirt, compared to the mass-produced garlic found in netted bags from big box stores which are smaller, dried, stark-white, less oily, and often imported from foreign countries such as China.

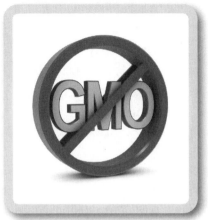

A few examples of information I learned from my local farmer's market store are as follows:

- **Burdock Root** – loaded with potassium; *helps your body make hormones which regulate your internal clock as well as your mood;* Burdock root is an excellent source of vitamin B6

- **Kukicha Twig Tea**[14]– rejuvenates your body from the inside out; alkalizes your body; infused with vitamins and minerals

- **Turmeric Root** – Curcumin, the active ingredient in turmeric has powerful antioxidant effects. It neutralizes free radicals on its own, then stimulates the body's own antioxidant enzymes. Turmeric may be the most effective nutritional supplement in existence. Many high-quality studies show that it has major benefits for your body and brain.

---

14   www.tinyurl.com/edenfoods-kukicha

> **The vegan lifestyle is not about feeding your stomach.Instead,it's about feeding your organs and system at a cellular level to create an environment of optimum health.**

In fact, a wonderful source of information about local farmers and an interesting array of chemical-, pesticide-, and GMO-free organic foods are available at your local organic store. While you make friends, you learn about life and they are happy to embrace you as new friends and a good customer.

There are many businesses like this out there, but we have seen them squished into the background by the advent of the big box stores, which are deemed one-stop-buys-everything; but there is a cost to that!! You don't get the variety or the personalized informed service that you do at the small businesses. There is a misconception that small business offerings are more expensive, but that's not true once you learn more and are more informed about your purchases, and what you are buying.

The vegan lifestyle is not about feeding your stomach. Instead, it's about feeding your organs and system at a cellular level to create an environment of optimum health. That is timeless, and forms the foundation for your whole body.

"If you struggle to pay the good farmer, just wait till you pay the pharmacy."

—SUZANNE MILES

*"Strive to keep toxins away from you so you
can not just survive but thrive."*

—SUZANNE MILES

To enjoy an empowered life with good health at the foundation of all you do is just the beginning of what you are capable of achieving. You may start a new business or write a book like I have. You may see a gap to fill, or an opportunity to buy a plot of land yourself and grow your own food. Maybe you'll develop a clothing or skin care line and sell to and help others.

We are chained or freed by our health condition. We all know that when we are not well, we lose our power. We can't go to work or go out and play, so let's remember this and make your health a priority.

*"If you keep good food in your fridge,
You will eat good food."*

— ERRICK MCADAMS

71

Grapes

Almond Butter

Kiwi Fruit

Squash

Pineapple

Lifestyle

Almond Milk Cabbage

Bay Leaf

Almonds Figs Flax seed Sesame Seeds

Apple Cider Vinegar Smoothies

Apples Maca Chlorella Cacao

Acai Spirulina Kale Brazil nuts

Strawberries

Gluten Free Healing

Green Tea

GREAT Blueberries

Ginger

DISCONNECT

Mango Lemons Green Juices

Garlic Turmeric

Tomatoes Bok Choy

Arugula Sunflower Seeds

Superfoods NON GMO Lentils

Kidney Beans Hemp Hearts

Baking Soda Black Pepper Himalayan Salt

Avocado Alkaline

72

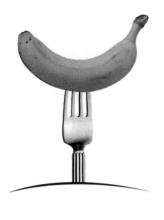

CHAPTER 8

The Great Disconnect

*N*ow is a great time to do a quick comparison of how your eating used to be, compared to now.

Take me, for example: Before becoming vegan, typically in the morning upon waking, the first thing I reach for was coffee, which I always added cream and sugar to. My husband left before me and had the coffee ready, and had already taken his. Perhaps I even had coffee at home, then picked one up on the way to work. The West Coast style of where I live is the drive-through coffee shop, double cream, double sugar, and you're on your way, feeling good. So that's the first daily double. Shortly after morning coffee, I may have reached for most commonly cooked breakfast, for example pancakes, bacon and eggs, croissant with ham and cheese, boxed cereals with milks, porridge in winter topped with brown sugar, or if in a hurry, muffins and donuts.

Then there's coffee breaks at work, which typically meant going out to get coffee with your workmates, again with more cream and sugar. Between noon and 1:00 p.m. would be lunch, which commonly was a sandwich with bread, ham and cheese, or tuna, egg, or chicken salad sandwich. Subway-style deli bun items perhaps, with the special deal of a pre-made soup style and a cookie. Then there's McDonald's, and all the fast-foods that we've all sampled at some point in our lives.

This all seemed quite right!! Because it was the same as it ever was since I was going to school as a child since I can remember. Oh sure, we switched from white bread to whole wheat bread thinking this was good.

Perhaps then even another pick-me-up sweet of some sort like chocolate, cookies, donuts, and another coffee with cream and sugar. You know how it goes!!

Then comes dinner. You're home after a day at work, kids are hungry, you're busy, and now dinner was normally comprised of meat such as chicken or fish, with a potato/vegetable combo of sorts. Perhaps even a Kraft dinner or a frozen, pre-made dinner plate. Weekends, perhaps, I may have made a roast of some sort of meat such as chicken, beef, lamb, or turkey. All these required lots of preparation, seasoning, and lots of garbage and cleanup. We always thought we'd use the leftovers, but as even you know, it rarely happens so it gets thrown out.

Let us now compare the above old eating lifestyle to the new lifestyle we enjoy so much more.

Up in the morning, and the first thing I reach for is a glass of water, followed by warm water with lemon cayenne. My husband and I both do this, however, now instead of leaving me coffee, he leaves a warm lemon drink. I love him for this; it's a kind act to start my day. Shortly thereafter, breakfast is now a blended fruit juice or smoothie, green and lean, filled with antioxidants, sustaining power for energy, and lots of fibre for good health.

Coffee break at work now is green tea or a tea that I create from loose leaves such as chamomile, mint, licorice, orange peel, and goji berry. Also, throughout the day loads of water, water, water, water, water! ☺

The old way of lunch is out the door! These days I tend to be able to glide through the work day on the morning drinks, and I pack myself a jar of dried fruits such as mulberries, cranberries, figs, prunes, and dates, along with some nuts and seeds like sunflower, pumpkin, cashew, Brazil, and almond.

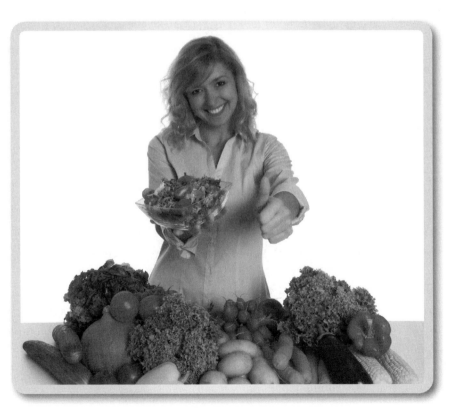

Dinner now is usually, depending on seasons, very easy in many ways. I can quickly make a big pot of medicinal soup, or my husband makes an amazing salad with fresh-cut vegetables and fruits, and placed on a board with some nuts and seeds. In medicinal soup I used foods like chickpea miso with dried maitake mushrooms[15], some chopped-up lever (seaweed), black pepper, kale, root vegetables, including garlic and ginger, plus som'e lentils for protein. Hot soup in the winter, fresh salads in the summer. Good fats from avocados, hemp hearts, and hemp oil, flax, sesame seeds and their oils. This is a loving way to eat.

> **Being vegan is a lifestyle that teaches you about yourself, and is a very giving and kind way of living.**

The gifts of eating vegan are not just about your body. It becomes a much deeper, grateful process. Yes, you may have to go through some bumps, twists, and turns, but upon pushing through the challenges and staying with the discipline, the gifts appear. Being vegan is a lifestyle that teaches you about yourself, and is a very giving and kind way of living.

After dinner, commonly I'll have my second cup of warm lemon water or a lovely herbal tea, perhaps peppermint and water.

Is it any wonder that my body is now feeling terrific? The previous eating style included high fat, over-portioned, oily and greasy, high sugar, chemically laden food that only satisfied an immediate need adhering to the ways of a system that is disconnected from your health. I was like a robot disconnected from the truth about food, eating mostly for taste and convenience rather than truly stepping up to the healthy plate. Is it any wonder we have a health crisis?

---

15   www.tinyurl.com/cancertreatment-mushroom

In combination with daily cardiovascular exercise, isn't it great that the body has the ability to respond in a very positive way?

It's very exciting and motivating to start seeing positive results from your efforts and the changes you've been making, including but not limited to weight loss (even two pounds is a great start). You start to look at your clothes and want to throw them out and get some new ones. You have improved energy, cleaner skin, your overall vibration is cleaner and lighter. You may even be meeting new people and making new friends. Keep going!!

The old way of eating was filled with animal fats, empty calories, chemicals, gluten, processed sugars, pesticides/herbicides, and GMOs. The new way is filled with antioxidants, fresh vegetables and fruits, organic produce, natural sugars, vitamins and minerals, protein from plants, nuts, and seeds, and offers much more than just the food. Your whole shopping experience changes. You become much more engaged with your kitchen; indeed, you find yourself cooking again. This is why it becomes a lifestyle. This is why we call it a plant-based lifestyle, as it connects into many parts of your life and reignites you from an almost dormant state of regularity built on a lifetime of being disconnected.

One of the things I did, and it's a work in progress, is that I changed the way the kitchen functioned. Now this isn't a big deal; it's a wonderful opportunity. Taking stock of what we needed and how we ate was and still is a fun and interesting experience. One of the first things I did was exchange the microwave (yes, we've lived without one in our home since 2011) for a juicer, for example. You can easily find all kinds of cooking items, including blenders and juicers, at thrift stores or yard sales. It doesn't have to be expensive to do a good job for you.

It doesn't take much to look back into your own family tree or the history books anywhere to see that the food prior to the 1950s was very different to the food today at this writing in 2014. People weren't eating fast-food. Everything was cooked at home, and people had food gardens and freezers. Things really changed in the '60s when fast-food places started to pop up, along with the music culture. Businesspeople and industrialists started to be much more involved in the production of food, purely for profit. This was, of course, the era of the Baby Boomers. Mass production of certain items started to become profitable, so suddenly, fast-food retailers started to spring

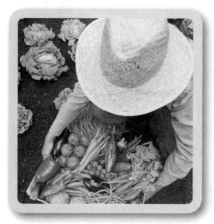

up in every neighborhood. This was marketed to our parents as a source of freedom. Freedom from cooking, and inexpensive to buy. It was marketed to the children as fun. That concept really took hold in that era, and paved the way to ill health for a few generations now. It shows no signs of slowing down as the industrialization of food has taken over everything.

The documentary *King Corn*[16] talks about the government-subsidized industrialization of food production. How at the time, the mandate of the day was to reduce the price of food.

Before the invention of condominiums, people lived in homes. Many homes had gardens, and a lot of our parents knew about food. Food was costly when I grew up in the '60s and '70s, with approximately 40% of income used by the food budget. This forged the development of food clubs, food stamps, big freezers separate from

---

16   www.imdb.com/title/tt1112115

the fridge, and it was instilled upon us to eat it all, everything that was on your plate, because food was a precious, expensive commodity. At the time we thought our parents were crazy and unfair, but parents of my generation had come out of the Second World War where food was rationed. So after the war and the immigration that occurred to America, Canada, Australia, and around the world, these people, our parents and grandparents, brought this knowledge about how precious food was. They were more connected than we are today.

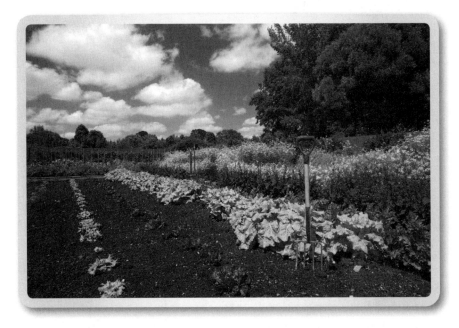

I have found that being a vegan has brought me a discerning attitude towards purchasing and consuming food. One discerning fact that I've come to know is that dairy products are poor sources of iron, and inhibit iron absorption. It's easy to build iron-rich blood being vegetarian or vegan; you replace meat with beans, peas, and lentils. Other good iron sources are nuts and seeds, especially pine nut and pumpkin seeds, dried fruits, blackstrap molasses, mushrooms, and grains. Quinoa is an excellent iron grain. To boost iron absorption, eat Vitamin C-rich foods.

Remember in your new kitchen to store your grains, spices, dried herbs, dehydrated fruits, nuts, and seeds in glass jars, preferably with lids and labeled. It's amazing how the most unorganized can get organized with this.

I have found that, over the years, I am always evolving. It's wonderful to be looking for new ways to achieve a cleaner, healthier, chemical-free life. It's a work in progress, and it's fun because you may plateau for a while, and suddenly you learn oh, I can clean my kitchen sink with a combination of baking soda, white vinegar, and lemon juice. If want to add a scent, I can put a few drops of tea tree oil, which is also antibacterial. This will make your kitchen sink, stove top, and bathroom shine. So now you are connecting more to the bigger picture of your involvement in the food system and the overall challenges facing the environment.

> So get connected and stay connected. Keep moving forward. It's a wonderful journey of enlightenment and empowerment. You get back in the driver's seat of your life.

"Dr. Dean Ornish, founder of the non-profit Preventive Medicine Research Institute, whose low fat almost vegan diet has been shown in one study to reverse arterial blockage, worries that an increase in animal protein consumption can come with health problems of its own, pointing to studies that link red meat in particular to higher rates of colon cancer. There's also an uncomfortable fact that meat, especially beef, has an outside impact on the planet. Nearly 1/3 of the earth's total ice-free surface is used one way or another to raise livestock. Even if eating more fat is better for us—which Ornish doesn't believe—it could carry serious environmental consequences if it leads to a major increase in meat consumption." (Quote from *Time Magazine*, June 23, 2014, written by Bryan Walsh, page 35.)

My body no longer goes through the peaks and valleys of the traditional lifestyle; the highs and the lows are gone. The 3:00 p.m. need for the sugar/caffeine energy boost disappears. This is all gone. Today I have a steady energy level that sustains me from dawn to dusk.

So get connected and stay connected. Keep moving forward. It's a wonderful journey of enlightenment and empowerment. You get back in the driver's seat of your life.

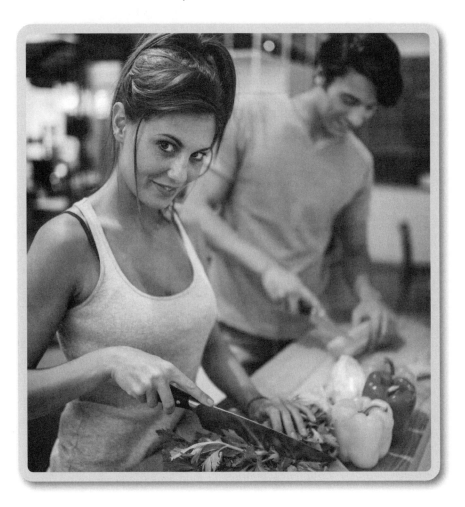

Mango Lemons
Garlic Turmeric
Tomatoes Bok Choy
Arugula Sunflower Seeds
Superfoods NON GMO Lentils
Kidney Beans
Hemp Hearts
Baking Soda Black Pepper Himalayan Salt
Avocado Alkaline
Green Tea
FOOD Blueberries
Ginger
MEDICINE
Kiwi Fruit
Almond Butter Squash Green Juices
Pineapple Lifestyle
Almond Milk Cabbage Bay Leaf
Almonds Figs Flax seed Sesame Seeds
Apple Cider Vinegar Maca Chlorella Cacao Smoothies
Apples
Acai Spirulina Kale Brazil nuts
Gluten Free Healing Strawberries
Grapes

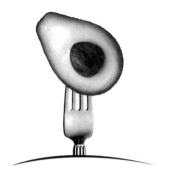

CHAPTER 9

Food Is Your Medicine; Medicine Is Your Food

Healing Herbs And Spices – Bring Them Into Your Kitchen And Into Your Life

*H*erbs and spices are so amazing. Many have been used for thousands of years. Some have direct health benefits while others add pizazz to your food; there's nothing like a hint of a hot spice to liven up a food plate. Many have detoxification properties, along with disease prevention benefits. Medicinally, many herbs and spices can cure illnesses and diseases, as Ayurveda healing would demonstrate.

This is a fascinating world of herbs and spices and a lengthy one—likely too long to list for this chapter. However, I want to touch on some that I know and use in my life for my body.

Herbs and spices not only assist in flavoring dishes and filling the air with delightful aromas, but they also hold medicinal properties that promote healing.

My number one herb has to be garlic. Garlic has been used for centuries for healing and warding off spirits. Organically grown, chemical-free garlic is what you want to source. Russian garlic or locally grown, organic garlic is often purple in color, in contrast to the stark-white ones you often find in supermarkets.

Good quality garlic is bursting with oil when you peel the skin back. The healing property of garlic is called allicin.[17]

Garlic – Helps fight infection, detoxifies the body, enhances immunity, lowers blood fats, assists healing of yeast infections, helps reduce asthma, cancer, sinusitis, circulatory problems, and heart conditions. Great for using in soups, salads, and enjoyed roasted. You can easily crush some garlic, mix with some apple cider vinegar and turmeric, and take as a daily shot of preventive wellness.

Turmeric - Turmeric grows wild in India. It has been used for over 2,500 years and is known for its purifying and healing benefits. Also known as curcumin, turmeric is increasingly recognized as a superfood that is used for the prevention of diseases and helps with skin problems. It is becoming well known, with a lot interest in turmeric for the prevention and slowing of Alzheimer's. It helps with cholesterol,

17   www.allicinfacts.com/about-allicin/what-is-allicin

improves digestion, and is a blood purifier, to name just a few of the many reasons everyone should take turmeric daily. Turmeric can be found in abundance, dried or fresh; it appears like a nob of ginger or a small carrot. You can easily grate or cut into pieces for soups and general eating.

A great way to take turmeric is to make a healing tea either in the morning, or as a calming tea before bed for a good night's sleep.

Ingredients

- 1 cup nut milk of choice, e.g., almond, rice, hemp, hazelnut, coconut
- 1/2 tsp turmeric
- 1 tsp cinnamon
- 1/4 tsp ginger

Directions

Heat the milk slowly on a stovetop (not microwave), stir in the spices. Enjoy!

Cayenne – An excellent spice added to a warm lemon water drink. Take it in the morning in replacement of coffee. Take it in the evening in replacement of tea and any caffeine. An excellent water-based drink to promote the alkaline body while offering the added healing properties of cayenne, including being a great metabolic booster. It aids the body in burning fat, controls blood sugar levels, reduces inflammation, and aids in detoxification. Fights colds and flu. Adds some pep to many dishes, including smoothies.

Ginger – This versatile root plant offers many amazing healing properties and can be easily taken as a tea, grated or chopped into salads, and even juiced. Ginger has long been used to help with motion sickness, helps with blood circulation, relieves menstrual cramps, and helps with digestion after meals. Ginger is well known for healing colds, coughs, and flu symptoms. Ginger in combination with turmeric and lemon can ward off the common cold through the winter months. It's an excellent all-rounder.

Rosemary – Grows wild as a woody shrub and offers a safe food supply for bees (so grow rosemary wherever you can). Rosemary has long been used as a reliever of headaches, as you can rub a few drops of the oil on your temples and forehead. Often, just sniffing the oil of rosemary offers a lift of mood and spirit. Rosemary is a powerful antioxidant, as the potent antioxidants within rosemary protect the body against free-radical damage. Rosemary is very good for alleviating stress. Rosemary is also known to improve memory, is anti-fungal, and anti-bacterial. Rosemary is excellent for your hair, helps you relax, and offers anti-aging properties. Women who are pregnant should avoid rosemary as it stimulates the body, so speak with your doctor before using rosemary. www.openhandweb.org/The_Amazing_Health_Benefits_ of_the_Humble_Herb_Rosemary

Cloves – These tiny but mighty nibs offer amazing properties when it comes to nutrition and natural health. They are native to the Maluku Islands in **Indonesia**, and are commonly used as a spice. Cloves are rich in antioxidants and antiseptic qualities, making them favorable as a healing spice. They are most widely known to assist with toothaches; however, these tiny giants also help boost the immune system and relieve digestive problems, as well as being an effective cure for wounds, burns, and bruises. I have grown to be able to munch on cloves much like you would a carrot. They are surprisingly easy to simply eat as part of a bag of nuts and seeds you may take hiking, for example. I also pop whole cloves into soups that I make, for added power.

Cumin – These powerful little seeds help control blood sugar, boosts the immune system, are great for keeping the skin looking youthful and vibrant, stimulate hair growth, help combat fatigue, and boost energy. They are used as a cancer fighter, and are high in antioxidants and antiseptic properties. Great for kidney health and promoting cardiovascular health. You use cumin as a powder or purchase the seeds, which are great to add into soups and salads. We use cumin with crushed red kidney beans and gluten-free tamari to make our own salt-free re-fried beans for tacos. Usually you will find pre-made refried beans out of the can to be very high in salt.

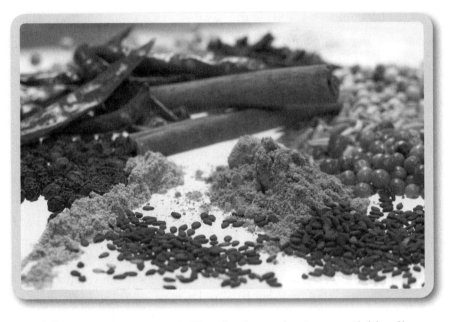

There are so many excellent herbs and spices available all over the world, so go exploring the world of herbs and spices. They bring beauty, health, scents, and joy into your life and cooking experiences. Use them widely, and take them often. Make these beauties part of your daily life.

The world of medicinal herbs and spices as mentioned above is extensive; the ones I've listed above you probably know of and use. There are many others I use that are leaning more into the medicinal properties of disease prevention versus the ones you know for everyday use. These include:

Burdock Root[18] - An excellent liver tonic, removes toxins and waste buildup in the blood. Loaded with iron and phosphorus. Offers numerous enzymes for the digestive tract, which is essential for breaking down and absorbing nutrients. Good for kidneys and digestive system, skin and scalp. Make as a tea, or chop and put into soups and salads.

Dandelion Leaf[19] - An abundant green source right in your backyard, packed with calcium, fiber, potassium, beta-carotene, and vitamin A. Dandelion is well known to help the liver, and is widely used as a detoxification tonic for liver, kidney, and bladder. The leaves of dandelion are excellent when juiced, or used chopped into salads or soups. Dandelion is one of those backyard wonders that is seeing resurgence in use for its healing and health-giving properties. The flowers of the dandelion are healthy as well, and look very pretty in salads or as a plate decoration. You can enjoy an excellent cup of dandelion tea any time of the day.

Milk Thistle - Milk thistle is an herb in the daisy family that has been used for more than 2,000 years in ancient medicine. Milk thistle is still used around the world for healing. Milk thistle is commonly known as a weed, however, in recent years, milk thistle is gaining in popularity as a healing tonic that is beneficial for the liver, kidneys, gallbladder, and the body. "In our toxic world there is a real problem for us when free radicals

---

18   www.tinyurl.com/benefit-of-burdock-roots
19   www.tinyurl.com/benefits-of-dandelion-root

are created by something other than natural metabolism. Breathing smoke, smog, pollution and more will cause the body to spawn free radicals. These atoms cause massive chain reactions that lead to cell mutation and cell death, which in turn can cause a ripe area for disease such as cancer to form. So it's apparent protecting cells from having their atoms turn into free radicals and turning free radicals back into stable atoms is a good thing." (Excerpt from www.HappyMothering.com)

Milk thistle is used as a preventative and protective plant of antioxidants. The active ingredient in milk thistle is a powerful antioxidant called silymarin, which not only helps protect against free radical damage, but also stimulates the repair of liver tissue. Milk thistle flowers, leaves, stalks, and roots can be eaten, turned into tea, cooked into a stew, or juiced. The easiest way for most people to take milk thistle is through a capsule form.

Nettle Leaf - Great for coughs and colds, it boosts the immune system, supports the nervous system, and strengthens the urinary tract. Use as a warming tea anytime you need a boost. Great for allergies and asthma too.

Red Clover - Another plant that likely grows in your backyard. Studies have shown the tea to be of benefit to alleviate symptoms of menopause. It's an excellent blood cleanser. Red clover is a great detoxifier, getting rid of heavy metals and toxins from your body. Commonly used as tea.

Yellow Dock Root[20] - In traditional herbal medicine, yellow dock is thought to be a general health tonic.

Yellow dock is thought to benefit the digestive tract, liver, and skin. One of its primary uses by herbalists is for skin conditions associated with poor digestion, poor liver

---

20   www.tinyurl.com/yellow-dock-remedies

function, or "toxicity." Like dandelion and burdock roots, yellow dock roots and preparations are used to improve conditions related to a sluggish digestive system, such as liver dysfunction, acne, headaches, and constipation. Because it improves absorption of nutrients, yellow dock is used to treat anemia and poor hair, fingernail, and skin quality.

Ashwagandha[21] - Is a revered Ayurvedic medicinal botanical. "Ashwagandha (*Withania somnifera*; also called Indian ginseng or Winter Cherry) is a medicinal botanical grown in India that is revered for the multiple, health-providing benefits of powders and extracts made from its roots and leaves. It has been used for thousands of years in Ayurvedic medicine as a daily tonic to help treat such psychological and physical ailments as stress, strain, fatigue, cognitive function, exercise recovery, inflammation, immune health, blood sugar balance, and cardiovascular health. In the past decade its use as a dietary supplement has become increasingly popular, particularly in the areas of stress reduction, energy, and mental cognition. Consumers recognize that daily consumption of Ashwagandha helps enhance well-being and the ability to better cope with stress and other negative consequences of modern lifestyles."

Lemon Balm - From the mint family, easily grown, this wide-leafed beauty makes an excellent tea or addition to a salad. Lemon balm is known to help with problems associated with anxiety, nervousness, and insomnia while detoxifying the body, combating bad breath, and boosting energy. Lemon balm is a wonderful herb with a soft scent. Restorative. Leaves you feeling warm inside. A wonderful, comforting herb.

---

21   www.sensoril.com/about-ashwagandha

In summary, I use a wide of variety of herbs and spices such as the above, and many more. There is something to learn from each of these plants, herbs, and spices. Arnica and comfrey are constants in my health cabinet along with Bach Flower Remedies (www.bachcentre.com/centre/remedies.htm) which are an amazing collection of healing tinctures from herbs all unto their own. I am a long-time user of these beauties.

It's interesting how we have mostly forgotten about the amazing healing properties of such plants, herbs, and spices. Indeed, during the '60s and '70s our parents were told to spray these plants because they were weeds. WOW! The industrial food system already had visions of how to take away backyard gardening and put us in their stores, all the while taking these healthy, healing foods away.

While it is best to source organic herbs and spices in the plant form, often you can also source these in capsules and powder form. Please be aware that many supplements use non-vegan fillers and GMO ingredients, including the capsule itself. Do look for products marked non-GMO and even gluten-free or certified organic.

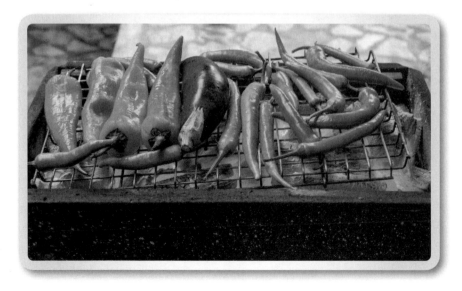

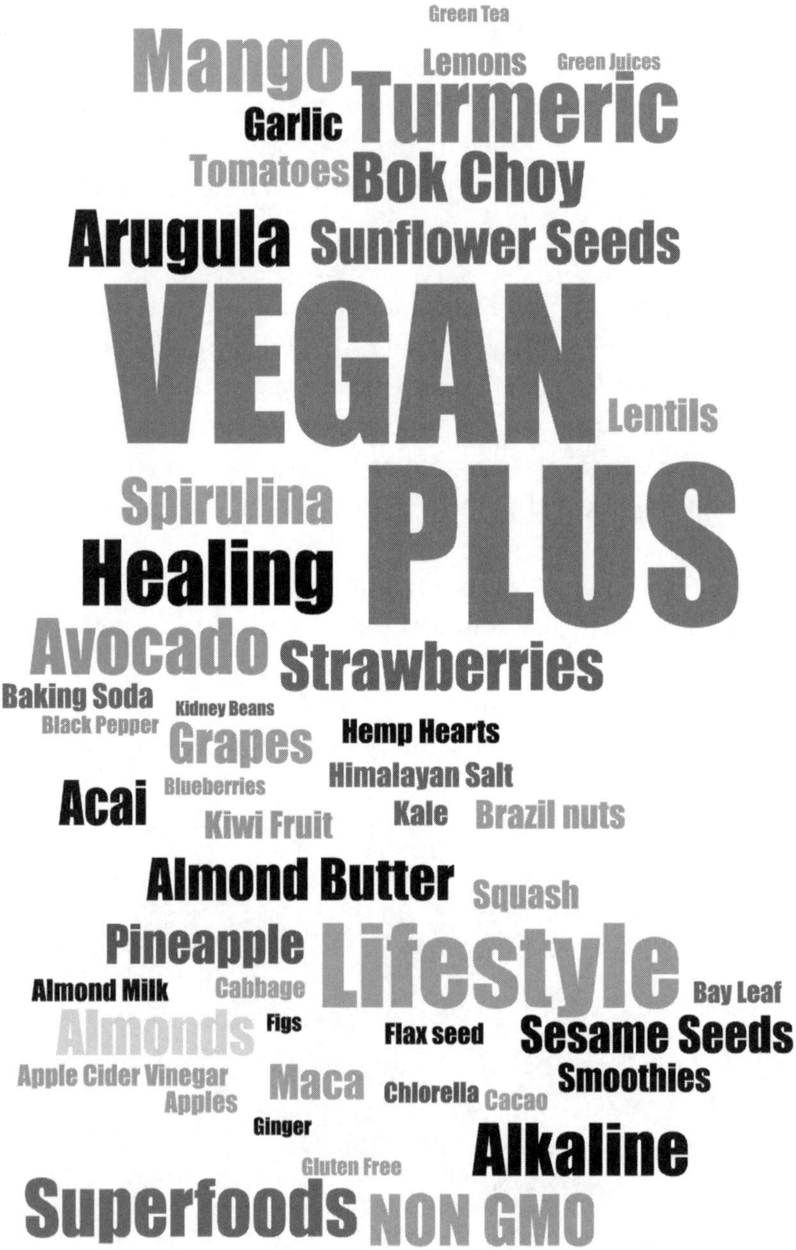

Green Tea

Mango Lemons Green Juices

Turmeric

Garlic

Tomatoes Bok Choy

Arugula Sunflower Seeds

VEGAN

Lentils

Spirulina PLUS

Healing

Avocado Strawberries

Baking Soda

Black Pepper Kidney Beans

Grapes Hemp Hearts

Himalayan Salt

Acai Blueberries

Kiwi Fruit Kale Brazil nuts

Almond Butter Squash

Pineapple Lifestyle

Almond Milk Cabbage Bay Leaf

Almonds Figs Flax seed Sesame Seeds

Apple Cider Vinegar Maca Smoothies

Apples Chlorella Cacao

Ginger Alkaline

Gluten Free

Superfoods NON GMO

92

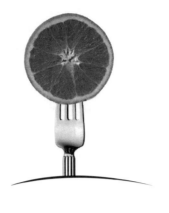

CHAPTER 10

Vegan Plus

To keep motivated and inspired with your new lifestyle, while continuing along the path you are on, it is important for you to amalgamate all the ideas shared with you in previous chapters, combined with what you already know at this point.

Always remember to include daily cardio exercise into your new lifestyle, and do your best to chart your results so you can see just how far you've come as time goes by.

It's also a good idea to have a complete physical and blood work done to be sure that your doctor is aware of what you are doing, and that you know exactly the starting point of your body's current state of health.

After all, the keys to amazing health is a pro-active approach. Take control. It's your body, it's your life. Enjoy a long and vital life. With good health, you are unstoppable. Join the centenarians! Go For the Glow!! www.facebook.com/pages/Go-For-Glow/122437757926951 Reach for a long and vital life; it's available to you.

> **Take control. It's your body, it's your life.**

As your body continues to cleanse, give it time to do its processing. Our organs and body are deep energy fields, and cleansing will take place immediately in fat loss. But in the longer term, your organs will eventually cleanse, and your body will detox the metals, toxins, and pollutants that are buried deep in you. You may notice the results of this cleansing with nicer hair texture, cleaner, clearer skin tone, acne goes away, wrinkles soften, and energy improves. Vitality returns to that of a person years younger. This is very exciting!!

Becoming more regular in your excrement is a very important sign of your health. Having to push to remove waste product is not a good sign of health. You will notice that your excrement changes a lot since starting a plant-based diet. Stools become softer, lighter, and easier to get rid of. Indeed, they just fall out quickly and easily.

It's a great idea to reward yourself for your newfound weight loss and improved energy with activities that are a lot of fun such as cycling, forest hiking, running, power walking, team sport activities, and generally engaging in the new body energy you have. It could be yoga, traveling...all kinds of things can come into play at this time for you.

Continue to motivate yourself by researching new food combinations, and investing in something new that applies to your lifestyle. Perhaps it's some new clothes, a new bicycle, a new blender or juicer; could be a trip you've always wanted to take.

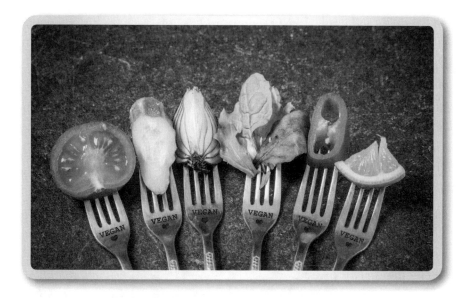

Another motivator I found to be very helpful was to seek and research other people who were doing what I am doing. I find this to be inspirational and motivating. Some high-profile vegans include Paul McCartney, Ellen DeGeneres, Bill Clinton, and Carlos Santana. I have also found others, such as the amazing Mimi Kirk [22] and Rich Roll[23]. Also Dr. Caldwell Esselstyn[24] and the recently new vegan, Dr. Sanjay Gupta[25] of CNN.

A great source of inspiration is to find local vegan restaurants in your town, or when visiting places that you travel to. Always source these places, as they could offer many ideas for you. Some are doing juicing, others smoothies. Others are full-on restaurants; some quite classy, others very grassroots. All have one thing in common—vegan health. That's what they sell.

---

22   www.youngonrawfood.com

23   www.richroll.com

24   www.dresselstyn.com/site

25   www.sanjayguptamd.blogs.cnn.com

One wonderful surprise you find when you go to a vegan restaurant is the price of the food. Many times entrées are under $10 because of the lack of animal products. One delightful dish I found very early in my vegan journey was a Portobella Mushroom Cap plate with a delicious cilantro sauce mixed with assorted vegetables. It was so delicious and tasty that after finishing it, we ordered it again. It was only $7!! How many times have you ordered the same entrée back to back because it tasted so good??? Think about it!!

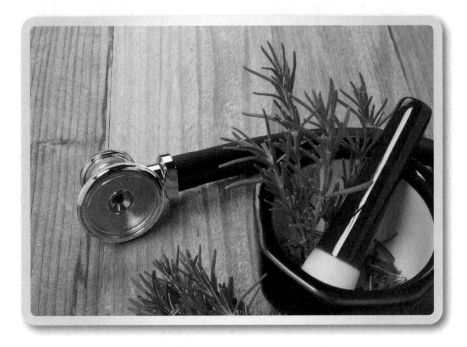

Continuing this culinary exploration will lead you to a world you don't even know exists, filled with interesting items of all kinds, and good people. You may find yourself at some vegan festivals around the world that are well attended, with the goal to share the amazing food gifts from the earth. The word of vegans is expansive beyond anything I even knew or experienced. And I thought I was doing pretty good on culinary knowledge.

After all, food is either your health, or your non-health. Your health is not so much formed by genetics as it is by food choices. You only need to turn on mainstream TV and learn that all the ads for food are paid for by fast-food companies, whereas you don't see healthy plant foods advertised for wellness. But you do see hamburger and fries with soda advertisements saturating TV.

> **Your health is not so much formed by genetics as it is by food choices.**

The vegan lifestyle is for every person on the planet, of all ages. From Mr. Universe to the new baby, everyone benefits from plant-based living. It's always a great inspiration to know that while living this lifestyle, your footprint on the world is one to be proud of, and one you can talk about and hopefully inspire others. You can sleep well knowing you are not contributing to climate change and global warming through being involved with the livestock and animal production industry.

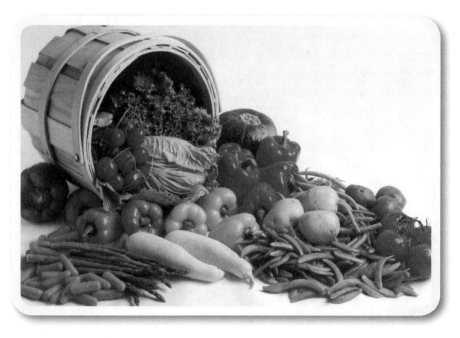

Personally I feel lighter, happier, healthier, and I'm always learning now. That learning will never stop. As you continue to learn about all the plants, herbs, and spices available, the learning of how to use them is huge. I am currently studying at the time of this writing about flower essences and the healing powers of flowers to our bodies.

The list of plants, herbs, and spices from the earth is far greater than the animals that have been pushed upon us to eat. Another investing motivator you can think about doing is to grow your own food, for example mint (in containers, or it will take over your yard), parsley, tomatoes, chives, garlic, and cilantro. Even on a windowsill in your New York apartment you can grow something! Whatever you grow, you know how it's been managed, which means chemical-free, pesticide-free, GMO-free clean food for you. Even on a small scale, it gets you involved in food—your food!!

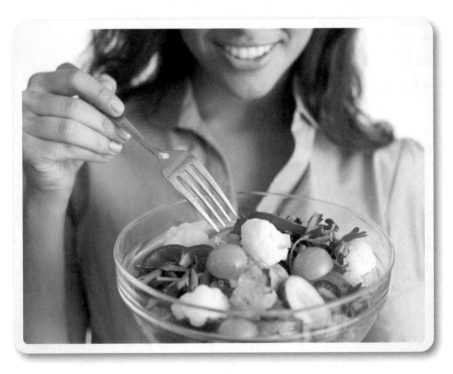

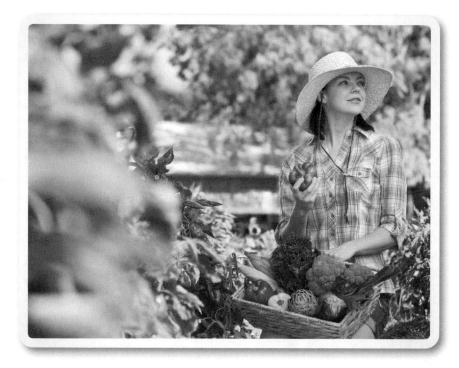

This is a very important juncture now, as I have learned that food has been pressed upon us by a system that actually does not have any interest in our health. It has one goal, and that's money. Peeling back the layers that you have been taught, to discover that you can have amazing health is very empowering, and a position all of us should employ.

No health, no wealth.

As the old saying goes, "No health, no wealth."

Today's informed consumers are no longer content to accept that all the additives and ingredients in foods, personal care, and cosmetic products are benign and therefore can do no harm. This increased awareness is building all the time as a result of personal experiences with illness and disease. These are rising as a health crisis in our modern-day society. Along with this is the proliferation of information available to us today that is exposing the damaging effects of many of the synthetic chemicals used for feeding animals and making products of all descriptions, including those used in foods and cosmetics.

My husband started a plant-based lifestyle at age 58. Here's a word from my husband: "I joined Suzanne right away, as I realized I needed this lifestyle as well. If she needed it and could benefit from it, why wouldn't I join in? At the time of this writing I am now 61 years young, and I've learned a thing or two about the misconception that men need meat. The concept that men need to eat meat because meat has protein for men is false. It is a fact that there is more than plenty of protein to get in a plant-based diet, and most meat-eating men have too much protein in their diet anyway. In my experience, for every meat flavor I thought I would miss greatly I have found

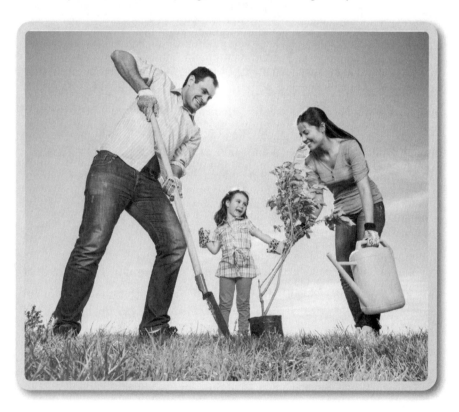

amazing substitutes which easily replaced and superseded any desire for me to want to reach for meat again. I have also learned about the hazards of meat, dairy, wheat, chicken—all that stuff. At 58 years old I was 50 pounds overweight, with high, pre-medication levels of blood pressure and cholesterol. I was prematurely aging, balding, with body flab, and who knows what other problems were quickly around the corner.

Now, since 2011, I have lost the 50 pounds, and my blood pressure and cholesterol levels are in the normal range. My doctor told me I was in the top 1% of the all the males he sees, and I am in very good health. After having a complete physical and blood work done, I was said to be a 'model of health for my age.' I attribute all of this to a plant-based food lifestyle and regular cardiovascular exercise. My culinary journey has been amazing, with more gifts than I expected. My relationship with my wife, the author of this book, has strengthened. We are more flexible and adaptable, and definitely happier as we enjoy the rewards of our lifestyle choice."

> **The ultimate goal is to have all the elements of your life working in synergy for your happiness so you can enjoy a long, grateful, fulfilled life.**

It's very important to the health of our bodies to understand that each chapter of this book will help you control and regain the most important thing in your life, the health of your body, mind, and spirit. We will gain a sense of freedom. At the same time, we can give back to the world a clean, green footprint to be proud of. Remember that the plant-based lifestyle should be kept in combination with daily cardiovascular exercise to have maximum effect. And a reminder—not all vegans are healthy vegans!! The ultimate goal is to have all the elements of your life working in synergy for your happiness so you can enjoy a long, grateful, fulfilled life. We must all work towards a chemical-free, sugar-free, animal-free, pesticide-free, GMO-free, gluten-free, alkaline body.

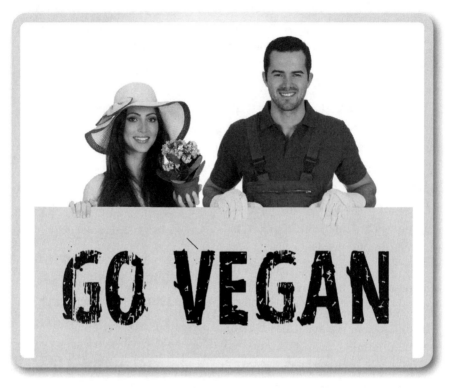

The keys to amazing health as outlined in the chapters in this book have come from our own experiences, tried and true. There have been many changes as we constantly moved forward in the lifestyle, letting go to move forward, so to speak. Much research has been done, and many facts have been learned. Temptations become less and less desired as other options become more appetizing, interesting, and available. It's an easy transition—not a hard one. The difficulties come from society; social and family pressures. But you will always be rewarded in the proof of yourself when people say to you, "You look so great, what are you doing?" It's right there that you know you have found something wonderful.

If you've read this book and in your vegan travels you see us, please say hello. We'd love to meet you!

Have fun with your vegan, plant-based journey. I wish you continued success in your health, longevity, vitality, and experiences that you enjoy in your life.

I hope I have informed, inspired and motivated you! May you take the plant-based lifestyle and aspire to motivate others.

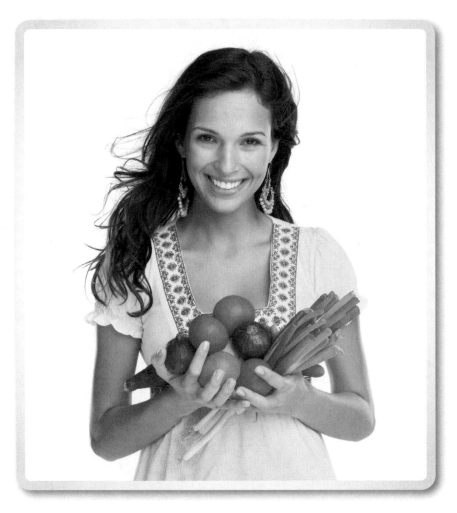

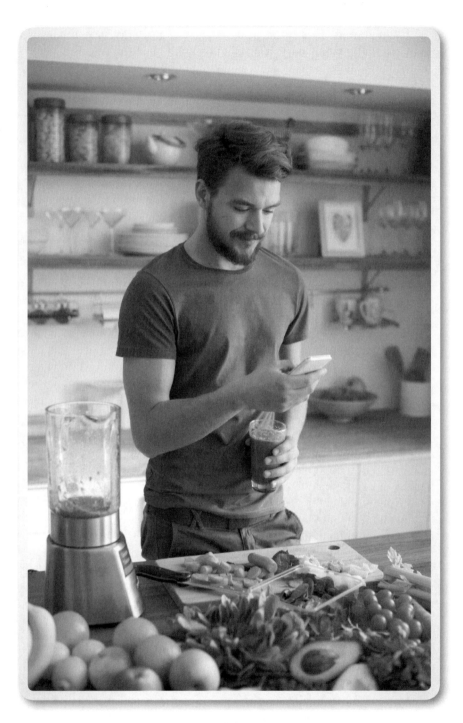

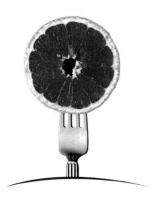

Testimonials

"Suzanne Miles has gone through an incredible evolution of Body, Mind and Spirit. Through her inspired journey she brings the essence of all the shifts that will bring you into a new path of joy, fulfillment and personal growth. What magnificent gifts Suzanne has to share with you"

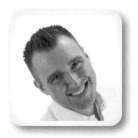

Lars Gustafsson
Founder: BodyMind Institute
www.bodymindinstitute.com/faculty/lars-gustafsson

"We had the privilege of having Suzanne in for a {modern glam} experience to create images for her upcoming book. Without having read a written word from her, but simply hearing her speak about the life-changing journey she and her husband had begun, my family and I were inspired to start our own lifestyle change and are already feeling the results in surprising ways! Thank you for sharing this with the world!"

"Everyone is beautiful and everyone deserves to see themselves that way!"

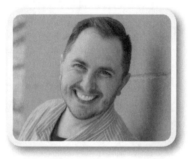

Tobin Smith - Portrait Photographer
photobin photography | 778.835.1203
www.photobinphotography.com
fb.com/photobinphotography

Scan this QR code to send an email to
smiles00@live.com and get your
FREE 60-minute Go For Glow
consultation with the author.

LET ME HELP YOU
LETS WORK TOGETHER

International Speaker / Consultant / Author as seen at the National Achievers Congress in Sydney, Australia 2015 at the Tony Robbins/Nick Vujicic/Richard Branson events!

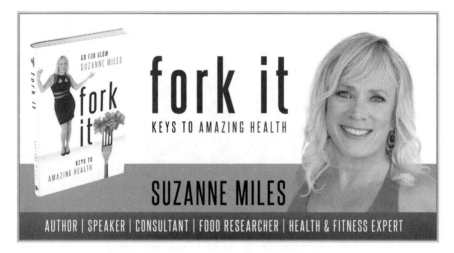

I offer information; inspiration and motivation on lifestyle, food choices and weight loss creating change opportunities to meet the demands of a new world.

- Motivational consulting on creating breakthrough results in your life.
- I offer speaking engagements and consultations for large groups, small groups, and private.
- Guest speaker at events; TV shows; radio talk ins; magazine interviews; newspaper articles; social media events and other opportunities.
- Consultant to businesses on best practices around health and lifestyle.
- Ongoing lifestyle coaching.

For all inquiries and bookingscontact me directly at:

Email Address: smiles0@live.com
Phone Number: 778.968.5470
Website: www.forkitbook.com
Facebook: www.facebook.com/suzannemilesforkitbook

Thank you,

Suzanne

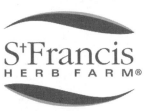
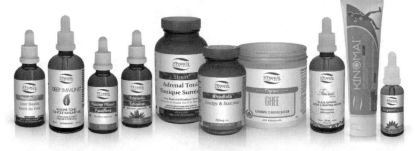

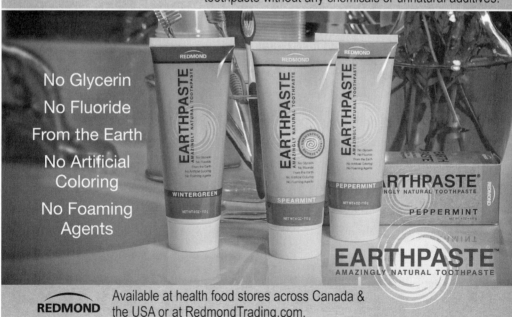   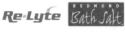

For all people committed to living a healthy life!

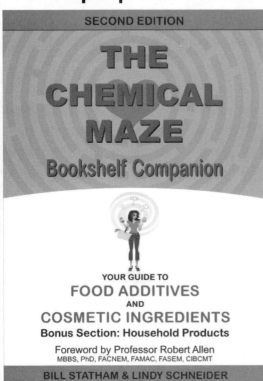
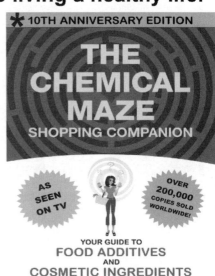
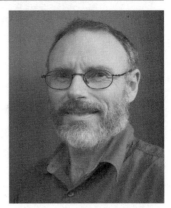

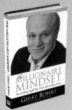
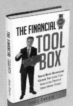
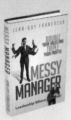
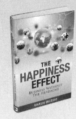
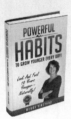
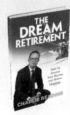
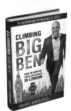
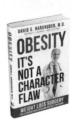

OTHER BOOKS RECOMMENDED BY BLACK CARD BOOKS

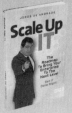

Scale Up IT
The Roadmap To Bring Your Enterprise To The Next Level
Jorge De Andrade

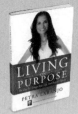

Living On Purpose
The Key To Change Your Life And Impact Others
Petra Laranjo

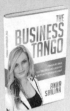

The Business Tango
Embracing Enterpreneurship & Intrapreneurship
Anna Shilina

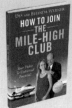

How To Join The Mile-Hign Club
Your Ticket To Unlimited Potential
Des and Belinda Werner

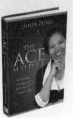

The Ace Model
Winning Formula For Audit Committees
Sindi Zilwa

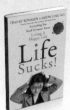

Life Sucks!
Everything You Need To Know About Living A Happy Life
Franky Ronaldy & Meow Ling Ng

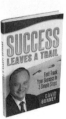

Success Leaves A Trail
Fast-Track Your Success In 3 Simple Steps
David Bunney

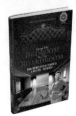

From The Bedroom To The Boardroom
How Women Can Be Powerful & Win Big - Anywhere!
Princess Tsakani Nkambule

www.blackcardbooks.com